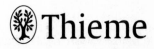

Abbreviations

ACE	angiotensin-converting enzyme	MEWDS	multiple evanescent white dot syndrome
ADOA	autosomal dominant optic atrophy		
AGEs	advanced glycation end products	MFERG	multifocal electroretinogram
AION	anterior ischemic optic neuropathy	MLF	medial longitudinal fasciculus
AMD	age-related macular degeneration	MRI	magnetic resonance imaging
ANA	antinuclear antibodies	NAION	nonarteritic anterior ischemic optic neuropathy
APMPPE	acute posterior multifocal placoid pigment epitheliopathy		
		NHL	non-Hodgkin lymphoma
ARC	anomalous retinal correspondence	NPDR	nonproliferative diabetic retinopathy
ARC	anomalous retinal correspondence	NRC	normal retinal correspondence
BRAO	branch retinal artery occlusion	NVD	neovascularization of the disk
BRVO	branch retinal vein occlusion	NVE	neovascularization elsewhere
cG	centigray	OAT	ornithine ketoaminotransferase
CHED	hereditary endothelial dystrophy	OCT	optical coherence tomography
CME	cystoid macular edema	OCT	optical coherence tomography
CNV	choroidal neovascularization	OKN	optokinetic nystagmus
CNV	choroidal neovascularization	p.o.	by mouth
CPEO	chronic progressive external ophthalmoplegia	PAS	periodic acid-Schiff
		PCP	Primary chronic polyarthritis
CRAO	central retinal artery occlusion	PDR	proliferative diabetic retinopathy
CRVO	central vein occlusion	PEX	pseudoexfoliation
CT	computed tomography	PHPV	persistent hyperplastic primary vitreous body
DAG	diacyl glycerol		
DR	diabetic retinopathy	PIC	punctate internal choriopathy
EDTA	ethylenediaminetetraacetic acid	PION	posterior ischemic optic neuropathy
EOG	electro-oculogram	PKC	protein kinase C
ERG	electroretinogram	PMMA	polymethylmethacrylate
ESR	erythrocyte sedimentation rate	POHS	presumed ocular histoplasmosis syndrome
FA	fluorescence angiography		
GVH	graft-versus-host reaction	PPRF	paramedian pontine reticular formation
Gy	gray [radiation unit]		
HE	hematoxylin and eosin	PPV	pars plana vitrectomy
HLA	human leukocyte antigen	PRK	photorefractive keratectomy
HPV	human papilloma viruses	PTC	pseudotumor cerebri
HSC	herpes simplex virus	PTT	partial thromboplastin time
ICE	iridocorneal endothelial	PVR	proliferative vitreoretinopathy
ICG	indocyanine green	RAPD	relative afferent pupillary defect
ICGA	indocyanine green angiography	RIMLF	rostral interstitial nucleus of the medial longitudinal fasciculus
INO	internuclear ophthalmoplegia		
INR	international normalized ratio	ROP	retrolental fibroplasia
IOL	intraocular lens	SLE	systemic lupus erythematosus
IRMA	intraretinal microvascular abnormality	t.i.d.	three times daily
ISNT	inferior > superior > nasal > temporal	TINU	tubulointerstitial nephritis and uveitis
LASEK	laser epithelial keratomileusis	TTT	transpupillary thermotherapy
LASIK	laser in situ keratomileusis	TPA	tissue plaminogen activator
LC	laser photocoagulation	UBM	ultrasonic biomicroscopy
LGB	lateral geniculate body	VEGF	vascular endothelial growth factor
LH test	Lea Hyvärinen test	VEP	visual evoked potential
LIPCOF	lid margin parallel conjunctival folds	VEP	visual evoked potentials
MALT	mucosa-associated lymphoid tissue	VOR	vestibulo-ocular reflex

Pocket Atlas of Ophthalmology

Torsten Schlote, MD
Associate Professor
Eberhard Karls University
Tuebingen University Eye Clinic
Ophthalmology I
Tuebingen, Germany

Matthias Grueb, MD
Eberhard Karls University
Tuebingen University Eye Clinic
Ophthalmology I
Tuebingen, Germany

Joerg Mielke, MD
Eberhard Karls University
Tuebingen University Eye Clinic
Ophthalmology II
Tuebingen, Germany

Jens Martin Rohrbach, MD
Professor
Eberhard Karls University
Tuebingen University Eye Clinic
Ophthalmology I
Tuebingen, Germany

With contributions by
Faik Gelisken, Matthias Grueb, Detlef Holland, Joerg Mielke,
Jens Martin Rohrbach, Torsten Schlote, Ulrike Schneider,
Hans-Sebastian Walter, Petra Weckerle

537 illustrations
40 tables

Georg Thieme Verlag
Stuttgart · New York

Library of Congress Cataloging-in-Publication Data

Pocket atlas of ophthalmology / edited by Torsten Schlote... [et al.]; with articles by Faik Gelisken ... [et al.].
p. ; cm.
Includes bibliographical references and index.
ISBN 3-13-139821-3 (GTV: alk. paper) –
ISBN 1-58890-452-0 (TNY: alk. paper)
1. Ophthalmology–Atlases. 2. Eye–Diseases–Atlases. I. Schlote, Torsten. II. Gelisken, Faik. III. Title. [DNLM: 1. Eye Diseases–Atlases.
WW 17 P739 2006a]
RE71.P64 2006
617.7–dc22

2006011949

This book is an authorized and revised translation of the 1st German edition published and copyrighted 2004 by Georg Thieme Verlag, Stuttgart, Germany. Title of the German edition: Taschenatlas Augenheilkunde

Translator: mt-g Medical Translation GmbH, Neu-Ulm, Germany

© 2006 Georg Thieme Verlag,
Rüdigerstrasse 14, 70469 Stuttgart, Germany
http://www.thieme.de
Thieme New York, 333 Seventh Avenue,
New York, NY 10001, USA
http://www.thieme.com

Cover design: Thieme Marketing
Drawings: Karin Baum
Typesetting by OADF Electronic Publishing, Holzgerlingen
Printed in Germany by Appl Aprinta Druck, Wemding

10 ISBN 3-13-139821-3 (GTV)
13 ISBN 978-3-13-139821-5 (GTV)
10 ISBN 1-58890-452-0 (TNY)
13 ISBN 978-1-58890-452-2 (TNY)

1 2 3 4 5 6

Important note: Medicine is an ever-changing science undergoing continual development. Research and clinical experience are continually expanding our knowledge, in particular our knowledge of proper treatment and drug therapy. Insofar as this book mentions any dosage or application, readers may rest assured that the authors, editors, and publishers have made every effort to ensure that such references are in accordance with **the state of knowledge at the time of production of the book**.

Nevertheless, this does not involve, imply, or express any guarantee or responsibility on the part of the publishers in respect to any dosage instructions and forms of applications stated in the book. **Every user is requested to examine carefully** the manufacturers' leaflets accompanying each drug and to check, if necessary in consultation with a physician or specialist, whether the dosage schedules mentioned therein or the contraindications stated by the manufacturers differ from the statements made in the present book. Such examination is particularly important with drugs that are either rarely used or have been newly released on the market. Every dosage schedule or every form of application used is entirely at the user's own risk and responsibility. The authors and publishers request every user to report to the publishers any discrepancies or inaccuracies noticed.

Preface

Like other medical specialties, ophthalmology undergoes constant enormous development in all its subspecialties. Assembling essential information is therefore an ever-recurring task, which needs to be done in various ways and for various target groups. The specialty of ophthalmology owes its development in recent years to numerous technical innovations. However, these can benefit the patient fully only when there is comprehensive knowledge of the clinical features of diseases. The primary concern of this pocket atlas is to assist with this.

A pocket atlas of ophthalmology does not and cannot compete with detailed textbooks. However, the special concept of the pocket atlas has permitted the inclusion of an extraordinarily wide range of illustrations as measured by the overall scope of the book. The up-to-date explanations in the text support these illustrations in a deliberately brief form, as the aim of all the authors involved was to integrate essential information about all the important diseases of the specialty.

The book is intended for students and junior doctors training in ophthalmology, without rendering detailed textbooks superfluous. However, the ready availability of basic information coupled with the extensive illustrations should awaken the interest of colleagues in other specialties.

At this point, the editors would like to thank all of the authors involved, who through their competent articles enabled the entire spectrum of the latest clinical ophthalmology to be illustrated in a compressed form. Our special thanks go to Ms. Regina Hofer, graphic artist at Tübingen University Eye Clinic, whose illustrations

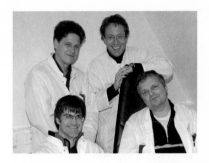

have substantially enriched this pocket atlas. Furthermore, we are greatly obliged to the staff of the photographic department of Tübingen University Eye Clinic as the majority of the high-quality illustrations is derived from their work and they assisted us actively in the choice of illustrations. We thank and acknowledge the publisher, Thieme, for not hesitating to turn this project into a reality in times of constricted economic scope. We also thank Randall L. Goodman, Santa Maria, California, USA, for his invaluable assistance in adapting the book to meet the needs of the international marketplace.

We hope and wish that this atlas will provide readers with a clearly structured and informative book that will assist them in their practical work for the benefit of patients.

Torsten Schlote
Matthias Grüb
Jörg Mielke
Martin Rohrbach

V

Addresses

Faik Gelisken, MD
Eberhard Karls University
Tuebingen University Eye Clinic
Ophthalmology I
Tuebingen, Germany

Matthias Grueb, MD
Eberhard Karls University
Tuebingen University Eye Clinic
Ophthalmology I
Tuebingen, Germany

Detlef Holland, MD
Kiel, Germany

Joerg Mielke, MD
Eberhard Karls University
Tuebingen University Eye Clinic
Ophthalmology II
Tuebingen, Germany

Jens Martin Rohrbach, MD
Professor
Eberhard Karls University
Tuebingen University Eye Clinic
Ophthalmology I
Tuebingen, Germany

Torsten Schlote, MD
Associate Professor
Eberhard Karls University
Tuebingen University Eye Clinic
Ophthalmology I
Tuebingen, Germany

Ulrike Schneider, MD
Associate Professor
University Eye Clinic
Basel, Switzerland

Hans-Sebastian Walter, MD
Department of Ophthalmology
Karlsruhe, Germany

Petra Weckerle, MD
Eberhard Karls University
Tuebingen University Eye Clinic
Ophthalmology II
Tuebingen, Germany

Contents

A. Eye

In addition to the eyeball **(bulbus oculi, A)**, the visual organ consists of the protective structures of the eye (orbit, lids, conjunctiva, and lacrimal apparatus) and the movement apparatus consisting of the extrinsic ocular muscles and Tenon's capsule. The optic nerve connects the sensory epithelium (the retina) with the brain. The eyeball is surrounded by the fatty tissue of the orbit.

B. Orbit

The frontal bone (orbital roof), zygomatic bone (lateral wall and floor), maxilla (floor), lacrimal bone and ethmoid bone (medial wall), and also the palatine bone and the sphenoid (blunt tip are involved in the structure of the orbit (**B**). The openings in the orbit are the optic canal (which contains the optic nerve), the superior and inferior orbital fissures, the infraorbital, ethmoidal, and zygomatico-orbital foramina, and the nasolacrimal canal.

C. Lids

The palpebral fissure is bounded by the upper and lower lids (**palpebrae**), the main structure of which is formed by a dense lid plate (tarsus). Exteriorly, the lids are covered by stratified keratinized squamous epithelium which becomes the palpebral conjunctiva at the lid margin. Lashes (**ciliae**) are found in 2 to 3 rows along the lid margin. The holocrine Zeis glands and the apocrine Moll glands end in the hair follicles. The excretory ducts of the larger Moll glands open close to the posterior lid margin. The eyebrow (**supercilium**) marks the upper border of the orbit. Blinking and closing of the lids is performed mainly by the orbicularis oculi muscle (innervated by the facial nerve). The levator palpebrae superioris (oculomotor nerve) and superior and inferior tarsal muscles (cervical sympathetic nerves) also open the lids. The sensory innervation of the upper lid is through branches of the first division of the trigeminal nerve (V_1), that of the lower lid by branches of the second division (V_2).

D. Conjunctiva

The conjunctiva covers the posterior surface of the upper and lower lids as the **palpebral conjunctiva**. It consists of two or more layers of isoprismatic – to highly prismatic epithelium. At the upper and lower fornix it changes to the **bulbar conjunctiva**, which is slightly mobile where it lies over the sclera. The conjunctiva consists of stratified nonkeratinizing epithelium.

E. Lacrimal Apparatus (E)

The lacrimal gland (**glandula lacrimalis**) lies above the outer corner of the eye. It is a tubuloalveolar gland whose 6–12 excretory ducts end in the lateral upper conjunctival fornix. The secretory parasympathetic innervation follows the facial nerve and the sympathetic innervation is through the cervical sympathetic. The tear fluid is low in protein and of low viscosity. Through blinking, the tears reach the medial angle of the lids and the fluid drawn into the lacrimal punctum and into the lacrimal canaliculi (**canaliculi lacrimales**). These open into the lacrimal sac (**saccus lacrimalis**) and from there the tears flow out through the nasolacrimal duct into the lower nasal passage (**E**).

F. Motor Apparatus

The extrinsic **ocular muscles** (2 horizontal, 2 vertical, and 2 oblique) lie in the fat of the orbit and move the eyeball. The superior, inferior, medial, and lateral rectus muscles originate from the tendinous ring, which forms the tip of the muscle pyramid at the orbital apex, and pass over the equator of the eyeball. With the exception of the lateral rectus muscle, which is innervated by the abducent nerve (CN VI), and the superior oblique muscle, which is innervated by the trochlear nerve (CN IV), they are innervated by the oculomotor nerve (CN III). The inferior oblique muscle arises from the medial wall of the orbit. The superior oblique muscle passes from the tendinous ring initially to the medial wall of the orbit, where it changes its direction at the trochlea.

A. Eye

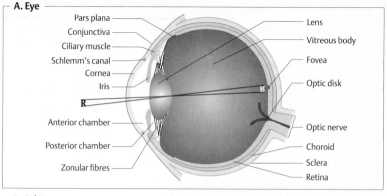

- Pars plana
- Conjunctiva
- Ciliary muscle
- Schlemm's canal
- Cornea
- Iris
- R
- Anterior chamber
- Posterior chamber
- Zonular fibres
- Lens
- Vitreous body
- Fovea
- Optic disk
- Optic nerve
- Choroid
- Sclera
- Retina

B. Orbit

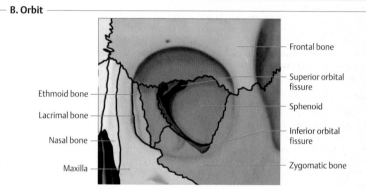

- Ethmoid bone
- Lacrimal bone
- Nasal bone
- Maxilla
- Frontal bone
- Superior orbital fissure
- Sphenoid
- Inferior orbital fissure
- Zygomatic bone

E. Lacrimal Apparatus

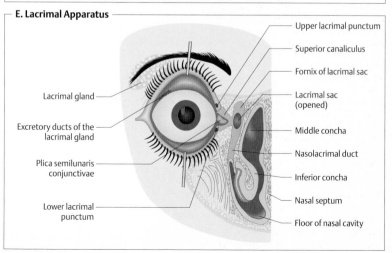

- Lacrimal gland
- Excretory ducts of the lacrimal gland
- Plica semilunaris conjunctivae
- Lower lacrimal punctum
- Upper lacrimal punctum
- Superior canaliculus
- Fornix of lacrimal sac
- Lacrimal sac (opened)
- Middle concha
- Nasolacrimal duct
- Inferior concha
- Nasal septum
- Floor of nasal cavity

A. Blood Supply

The **ophthalmic artery** is a branch of the internal carotid artery and passes into the orbit with the optic nerve. It then runs forward with the superior oblique muscle and ends as the dorsal nasal artery and supratrochlear artery. Before that it gives off the following branches: the central retinal artery, which travels to the retina in the optic nerve (**A**); short and long posterior ciliary arteries to the choroid and ciliary body; the lacrimal artery to the lacrimal gland; the supraorbital artery to the forehead; and the anterior and posterior ethmoidal arteries to the ethmoid air cells. The anterior ciliary arteries arise from the muscular branches to the extrinsic ocular muscles, which pass through the sclera to the ciliary body and iris. The **superior ophthalmic vein** collects the blood from the eyeball, upper orbit, lids and ethmoid air cells and drains into the cavernous sinus. The **inferior ophthalmic vein** arises on the floor of the orbit and flows either into the superior ophthalmic vein or into the pterygoid plexus.

B. Eyeball

The eyeball (**B**), **bulbus oculi**, has an almost spherical shape with an average diameter of 23 mm. The eyeball is bounded anteriorly by the cornea. At the posterior pole, the optic nerve leaves the eye somewhat medial to the axis of the eye, and the fovea centralis-which is the site of most acute vision-is somewhat lateral to this. The circumference at the greatest transverse diameter of the eye is called the equator. The wall of the eye consists of three layers: the outer layer (tunica fibrosa) with sclera and cornea; the middle layer (tunica vasculosa) with choroid, ciliary body, and iris; and the inner layer (tunica interna) with the retina and the retinal pigment epithelium. Inside the eye a distinction is made between the anterior and posterior chambers of the eye and the vitreous space. The cornea, aqueous humor, lens, and vitreous body constitute the optic media of the eye. The lens, zonular fibers, and ciliary muscle are called the accommodation apparatus.

C. Sclera

The sclera, which is white in adults, consists of packed lamellae of collagen fibers covering the posterior $5/6$ of the eye. At the corneal limbus it becomes the substantia propria corneae (stroma).

D. Cornea

The **cornea** has a diameter of about 12 mm in adults. The outside of the cornea consists of stratified nonkeratinized squamous epithelium, which changes to the epithelium of the bulbar conjunctiva at the corneal limbus. The inside is formed by a single layer of flat endothelial cells. Bowman's membrane is situated between the epithelium and stroma and Descemet's membrane between the endothelium and stroma (**Da**). The refractive power of the cornea is about 42 diopters (**Db**). The central thickness is approximately 500 μm.

E. Lens

The lens, with a horizontal diameter of about 10 mm, is situated in the posterior chamber of the eye. It is about 3–4 mm thick at the center. It is a biconvex lens, with the anterior surface less curved than the posterior surface. The lens shell, which surrounds the nucleus concentrically, lies beneath the lens capsule.

F. Vitreous Body

The vitreous body, which is 95 % water, fills the vitreous space situated behind the lens. Its gelatinous consistency is due to the presence of hyaluronic acid, mucopolysaccharides, and collagen fibrils.

G. Choroid

The choroid occupies the major part of the middle layer of the eye. In addition to arteries and veins, it also carries approximately 15–20 ciliary nerves. It is separated from the retina by Bruch's membrane, which is 2 μm thick.

A. Blood Supply

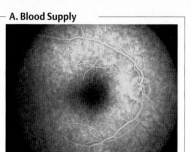

Angiography

B. Eyeball

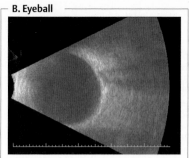

Ultrasound

D. Cornea

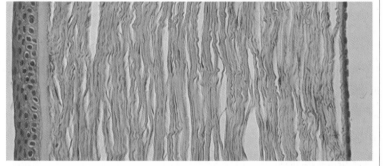

a PAS stain, ca. 63

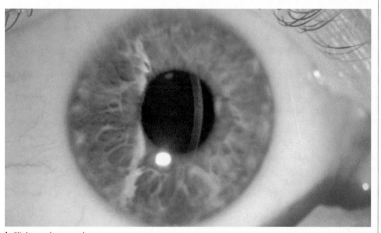

b Slit lamp photograph

A. Ciliary Body

The **ciliary body** (**Ba**) extends from the ora serrata as far as the base of the iris and surrounds the iris like a ring. A distinction is made between the outer part, the orbiculus ciliaris with fine meridional folds where the zonular fibers arise, and the inner part, the corona ciliaris. The ciliary body is covered by a bilaminar epithelium, which is responsible for the production of aqueous humor. The anterior and posterior chambers together contain about 0.2–0.3 ml of aqueous humor, most of which drains out at the iridocorneal angle. Part of the ciliary body is the ciliary muscle, whose smooth muscle fibers are arranged meridionally, circularly, and radially (parasympathetic innervation via the oculomotor nerve predominates with some cervical sympathetic input). Contraction of the muscle leads to slackening of the zonular fibers and, through the associated increased curvature of the lens, to accommodation.

B. Iris and Pupil

The iris, like a diaphragm, forms the **pupil**. The iris has no epithelium on its anterior aspect, so that the iris stroma, which is arranged radially to the edge of the pupil, is exposed. The iris is thinnest at the margin of the pupil and allows the bilaminar pigmented epithelium on the back to be seen. The pupil is surrounded by the sphincter pupillae muscle (parasympathetic innervation via the oculomotor nerve), the innervation of which produces contraction of the pupil (miosis). At the margin of the pupil, the iris is widely connected with the ciliary body. The muscle fibers of the dilatator pupillae muscle (cervical sympathetic) run here, contraction of which leads to pupil dilatation (mydriasis). At the **iridocorneal angle** (**Ba**), the aqueous humor flows through gaps in the pectinate ligament of the iris (**trabecular meshwork, Bb**) into Schlemm's canal.

C. Retina

The retina forms the inner layer of the eye. It is divided into a nonsensory part and an optic part, the boundary of which is formed by the ora serrata. The anterior part does not have any sensory epithelium and covers the ciliary body and iris as a bilaminar epithelium. The optic part consists of two layers, the outer layer (pigment layer) and the inner layer (cerebral layer), which lie loosely on one another and are adherent only at the ora serrata and at the entrance of the optic nerve. The central retinal artery and vein unite at the entrance of the optic nerve (optic disc or papilla). The macula lutea (yellow spot) is lateral to this with the fovea centralis at its center, the site of maximum visual acuity (**Ca**). The pigment layer consists of a single layer of isoprismatic epithelium (retinal pigment epithelium). The inner retina includes the photoreceptor cells and nine further identifiable layers of the cerebral layer (**Cb** and **c**). They are primary sensory epithelial cells. About 120 million rods and 6–7 million cones are distinguished. There are only cones in the fovea centralis, with no other layers of the cerebral layer. The perikarya of the bipolar cells, which are the second neuron of the optic nerve, are located in the inner nuclear layer. They maintain synaptic contact with the sensory cells in the outer plexiform layer and with the multipolar ganglion cells of the ganglion layer (third neuron) in the inner plexiform layer, from where sensory impulses are conducted in unmyelinated nerve fibers to the optic disc. The horizontal and amacrine cells of the inner nuclear layer form the association apparatus of the retina through the parallel connections of several synapses.

D. Optic Nerve and Optic Tract

The optic nerve is about 45 mm in length, two-thirds of which is inside the orbit. At the lamina cribrosa, ca. 1 million nerve fibers leave the eyeball and from this point are surrounded by a medullary sheath of oligodenroglia, dura mater and pia mater. After passing through the optic canal, it reaches the **optic chiasm** on the floor of the third ventricle after running about 10 mm in the middle cranial fossa. Here the nasal fibers of the retina cross to the opposite side. The optic nerve fibers run as the **optic tract** as far as the lateral geniculate body. The **optic radiation** (Gratiolet's radiating fibers) runs from here through the posterior crus of the internal capsule to the primary optic visual cortex, the **area striata**, area 17.

B. Iris and Pupil

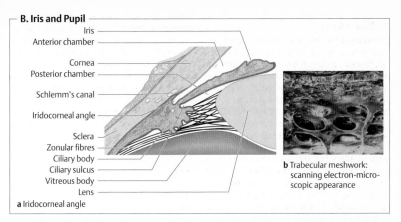

Iris
Anterior chamber
Cornea
Posterior chamber
Schlemm's canal
Iridocorneal angle
Sclera
Zonular fibres
Ciliary body
Ciliary sulcus
Vitreous body
Lens

a Iridocorneal angle

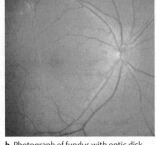

b Trabecular meshwork: scanning electron-microscopic appearance

C. Retina

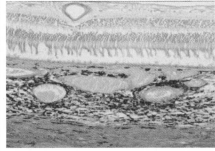

a Masson trichrome stain, ca. 150×

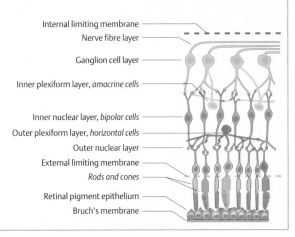

b Photograph of fundus with optic disk and macula

Internal limiting membrane
Nerve fibre layer
Ganglion cell layer
Inner plexiform layer, *amacrine cells*
Inner nuclear layer, *bipolar cells*
Outer plexiform layer, *horizontal cells*
Outer nuclear layer
External limiting membrane
Rods and cones
Retinal pigment epithelium
Bruch's membrane

c Diagram

A. Optical System

The light incident on the eye penetrates the tear film, cornea, aqueous humor, lens, and vitreous body, which constitute the optical system of the eye. Although the eye consists of several refractive components, for simplicity it can be compared to a simple lens system (**Aa** and **b**): light rays that pass from one medium (of refractive index n_1) into another medium (of refractive index n_2) are refracted. When the interface is simply convex, all the rays emerging from an object (O) meet again in an image (I) beyond the interface. The focal length, i. e. the distance of the focus (F_1/F_2) from the central plane of the lens system, is characteristic of a lens system. Rays that originate from a distant point can be regarded as parallel and they meet in the focal plane. Rays that originate from a near point do not arrive parallel and they form an image behind the focal plane.

B. Accommodation

Accommodation signifies the ability of the eye to **focus** the rays from objects to form a clear image on the retinal plane in relation to the objects' distance from the eye. Accommodation is based in particular on the ability of the elastic lens to change from a more spherical shape with high converging power (near focus) to a more elliptical shape with low converging power (distant focus). The passive tendency of the lens to adopt a spherical form is counteracted by the pull of the zonular fibers, which relax through contraction of the parasympathetically innervated ciliary muscle and so enable near accommodation to take place. In near focus this is accompanied by a bilateral convergent movement and miosis. The **converging power** is the *reciprocal* of the **focal distance** measured in meters. The unit of converging power is the diopter (D). The eye has a maximum converging power of ca. 58.8 D when accommodated for distant vision, and on maximum near accommodation this increases by about 10–15 D. This increase in converging power is called the **accommodation amplitude**.

C. Refraction Errors

As a result of increasing sclerosis of the lens and the associated reduction in accommodation power, the accommodation amplitude decreases with increasing age. This physiological event is called **presbyopia** (impairment of vision due to old age, **Ca, upper**). The near point moves increasingly into the distance. The patient notices a reduction in the ability to read from about the age of 45 years, when the accommodation amplitude falls below 3 D. Correction of presbyopia is through the use of a converging lens (+D).

In **myopia** (nearsightedness, **Ca, middle**) the parallel rays coming from infinity intersect in front of the retinal plane. The cause is excessive converging power of the cornea or lens (convergence myopia) or above-average length of the eyeball (axial myopia). The progressive malignant form of myopia must be distinguished from the simple benign form, which usually does not progress after puberty. Correction of myopia is through the use of a diverging lens (–D).

In **hyperopia** (farsightedness, **Ca, lower**) a point situated nearby is focused behind the retinal plane. Axial hyperopia, where the eyeball is too short, is distinguished from convergence hyperopia when the converging power of the cornea or lens is too low. Patients with latent hyperopia use their accommodation even with distant vision, which can lead to **asthenopic symptoms** (general ocular discomfort). Correction of hyperopia is through the use of a converging lens (+D).

The surface of the cornea is often more curved in one plane than in the other. The result is a difference in convergence in the two planes so that points appear linearly distorted. This regular astigmatism (**Cb** and **c**) can be corrected by cylindrical lenses. **Irregular astigmatism**, e. g., as a result of corneal scarring, can be compensated to a certain degree by hard contact lenses.

A. Optical System

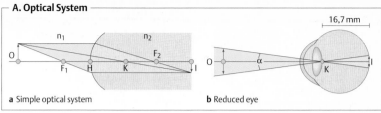

a Simple optical system

b Reduced eye

C. Refraction Errors

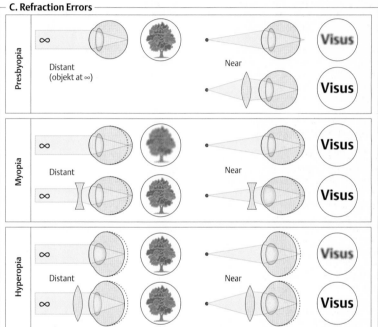

a Presbyopia/myopia/hyperopia

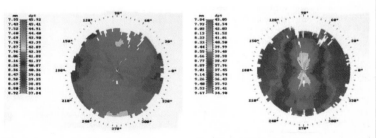

b Corneal topography with spherical cornea

c Corneal topography with astigmatic cornea

9

A. Visual Acuity

Vision in the eye relates to the overall function of the visual organ. Apart from pure visual acuity, it also includes the visual field, color vision, and dark vision. **Visual acuity** means the resolving ability of the eye with an optimally correcting lens, i.e. the ability of the retina barely to distinguish two points from one another (resolution threshold). A normal eye can just differentiate two points when the rays emerging from them form an angle at the eye of one minute of arc (1/60 degree). Visual acuity is calculated from the actual distance of the points from the eye divided by the distance at which the normal eye can resolve the points, and in the normal eye it is therefore $\frac{1}{1} = 1.0$. Optotypes projected into the distance (Landolt's rings, block letters, numbers, E hooks, children's pictures) or vision test tables for near vision (e.g., Birkhäuser tables) are used to test vision.

B. Receptors

Rods and cones constitute the retina's receptors. While the fovea centralis consists exclusively of **cones**, which are responsible for color vision in good lighting (photopic vision), their density diminishes rapidly toward the periphery. The **rods** are responsible for vision in poor light (scotopic vision); their greatest density is around the fovea centralis but they are also distributed over the entire retina (**Ba**). The photoreceptors are absent in the region of the optic disc. Under the effect of light, the **rhodopsin** located in the outer limbs of the rods and cones is bleached, leading to the conversion of light energy into electrical impulses through a change in the conformation of the pigment part from 11-*cis*- to all-*trans*-retinal (**Bb**). Rhodopsin is a chromoprotein and is a component of visual purple. It is composed of the protein opsin and the vitamin A derivatives 11-*cis*- and all-*trans*-retinal. In the dark, regeneration of the rhodopsin occurs with expenditure of energy. Absorption of light is required for the bleaching of the rhodopsin. As the rhodopsin contained in the rods absorbs light from the entire (visible) wavelength spectrum, different wavelengths (colors) cannot be distinguished by the rods. In contrast, the three visual pigments of the cones each absorb only light of a certain wavelength region, which allows for color vision.

C. Visual Field

The term **visual field** describes the area that is perceived at the same time when the eye is not moving. A distinction is made between monocular and binocular visual fields. The outer boundaries depend on adaptation and on the size, brightness, and color of the object and on whether the object is mobile or static. The boundaries are usually 60° nasally, 70° above, 80° below, and 90° temporally. The visual field is measured by **perimetry** (**C**). Two forms are distinguished:

- *Kinetic perimetry:* this records the site where a stimulus of defined brightness is first perceived as it is brought into the visual field.
- *Static perimetry:* measurement of the minimum brightness that a stimulus must have in order to be identified at a certain site with defined background brightness.

Defects in the visual field are called **scotomas** and can be symptoms of many eye diseases. The blind spot due to the absence of receptors in the optic disc is a physiological "scotoma." In the binocular visual field, each eye's blind spot is compensated by the other side. Temporally located objects are projected on the nasal half of the retina and vice versa. Objects in the upper visual field are imaged on the lower half of the retina, and objects from the lower region in the upper half of the retina.

B. Receptors

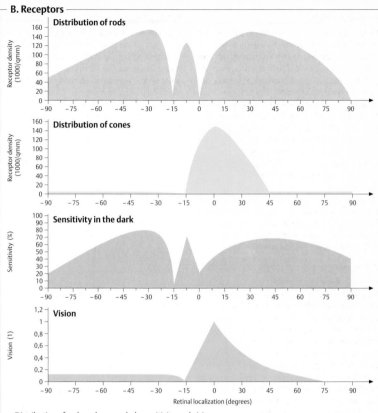

Distribution of rods

Receptor density (1000/qmm)

Distribution of cones

Receptor density (1000/qmm)

Sensitivity in the dark

Sensitivity (%)

Vision

Vision (1)

Retinal localization (degrees)

a Distribution of rods and cones, dark sensitivity and vision

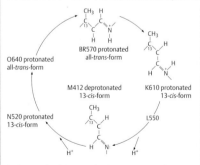

CH₃ H

BR570 protonated
all-*trans*-form

O640 protonated
all-*trans*-form

M412 deprotonated
13-*cis*-form

K610 protonated
13-*cis*-form

L550

N520 protonated
13-*cis*-form

H⁺   H⁺

b Photocycle of bacteriorhodopsin (BR): numbers
correspond to the wavelength of the absorption
maximum in nanometers

C. Visual Field

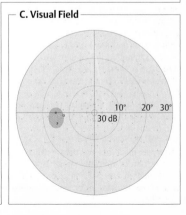

10° 20° 30°
30 dB

A. Adaptation

Adaptation (**A**) signifies the adjustment of the eye to different light levels. This is a complex process, which comprises a change in pupil size, a change between rod and cone vision, and a change in the sensitivity of the retina. According to the **duplicity theory of vision**, daytime and color vision (photopic vision) is a function of the cone apparatus, while vision in dim light and night vision (scotopic vision) are provided by the rod apparatus. **Light adaptation** means the transition to photopic vision and is based on pupil constriction and the transition from rod to cone vision with the breakdown of rhodopsin. The first phase of the transition (alpha adaptation) occurs in about 0.05 seconds, while the second phase (beta adaptation) lasts 6–7 minutes. The transition to scotopic vision (**dark adaptation**) takes place much more slowly and is complete after about 30 minutes. The first phase comprises cone adaptation and ends after about 7–8 minutes with the Kohlrausch notch, the transition to cone adaptation with the regeneration of rhodopsin. Dark adaptation is associated with pupil dilatation, a loss of color vision, a reduction in visual acuity, and a physiological central scotoma.

B. Color Vision

Color vision is a function of the cones. The wavelength spectrum of light perceived by the eye is between 400 nm and about 700 nm. According to the Young-Helmholtz three-color theory (**Bb**), three types of cones are distinguished: those that absorb blue-violet light, those that absorb green light, and those that absorb yellow-red light (the **trichromatic system, Ba**). According to the laws of color mixing, all other colors (including white) can be mixed from light of these three colors. The rhodopsin of the rods absorbs light from the entire visible wavelength spectrum, which is why it is not possible to distinguish colors with scotopic vision.

C. Central Processing

The stimulus of incident light leads to **hyperpolarization** of the primary membrane potential in the receptors of the retina. The magnitude of the potential increases with increase in the stimulus strength. When it crosses the threshold, this **secondary receptor potential** leads to **action potentials** in the corresponding ganglion cell, the frequency of which is proportional to the magnitude of the receptor potential. Through cross-connections within the retina (horizontal cells and amacrine cells), receptive fields occur that exert stimulating and inhibiting influences on the action potentials. Such a receptive field consists of a round center and a concentrically ordered periphery. If the light impulse falls on the center, the frequency of the action potentials rises. Illumination of the periphery leads to a fall in the action potential frequency. If the light stimulus is absent, excitation occurs in the peripheral part of the receptive field. Such a receptive field is called an ON field in contrast to an OFF field with the opposite reaction. The function of the receptive fields is to contrast the sensory stimulus.

D. Pupillary Reflex

The **pupillary reflex** is triggered by the sudden incidence of light into a pupil. The eye reacts with miosis (direct reaction). The contralateral pupil also contracts due to the central crossover of the stimulus (consensual reaction).

Afferent supply: optic nerve

Efferent supply: parasympathetic fibers via the oculomotor nerve.

E. Corneal Reflex

The **corneal reflex** is triggered by touching the cornea, which leads to reflex lid closure.

Afferent supply: trigeminal nerve

Efferent supply: mainly the facial nerve.

A. Adaptation

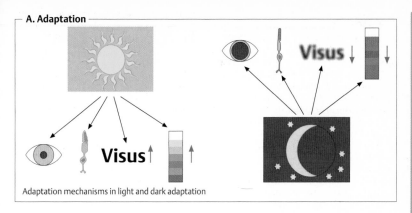

Adaptation mechanisms in light and dark adaptation

B. Color vision

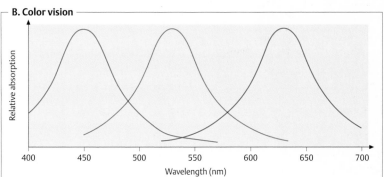

a Absorption spectra of the different cone types

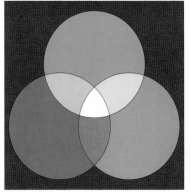

b Additive color vision: Young–Helmholtz three-color theory

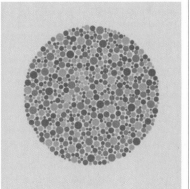

c Ishihara plate for testing color vision

A. Malformations and Anomalies

Microblepharon is vertical shortening of the lid fissure and ankyloblepharon means horizontal shortening as a result of adhesions of the lid margins. The temporal side is most commonly affected. Both changes are often associated with other anomalies of the eye or skin (**Aa** and **b**). **Cryptophthalmos** can be regarded as total ankyloblepharon, where the eye is completely covered by the skin of the forehead or cheek. In children, a thick skin fold running parallel to the lower lid margin (**epiblepharon, Ac**), which can induce astigmatism, or a crescent-shaped fold at the inner margin of the upper eyelid (**epicanthus, Ad**), which stretches from the upper to the lower lid and hides the canthus, is often found. This condition, also called a Mongolian fold, is occasionally associated with a slanted lid fissure and ptosis and can look like esotropia (pseudostrabismus). However, the corneal light reflections are parallel and adjusting movements are not present with cover testing. Epicanthus is found in about 30 % of all neonates and disappears by school age with the development of the nasal skeleton. Epicanthus is also often found in Down syndrome. **Telecanthus** designates an increased distance between the two canthi when the pupils are a normal distance apart. **Lid coloboma** means a unilateral or bilateral cleft, which usually affects the entire thickness of the lid. This is a rare, sporadic, congenital abnormality due to defective closure of the optic cup. **Polytrichosis** signifies the occurrence of incorrectly positioned individual lashes. In **distichiasis** an additional second row of lashes can be seen. Both diseases are rare congenital abnormalities of cellular differentiation. Besides sporadic cases, autosomal dominant inheritance has also been described. Lash anomalies are also found after trauma or with scarring dermatoses. Association with tarsal abnormalities, entropion, and narrowing or shortening of the lid fissure (**blepharophimosis**) is possible. The clinical significance is usually determined by the degree of trichiasis (misdirected lashes that irritate the ocular surface). Treatment of trichiasis can be performed with epilation, cryotherapy, laser coagulation or surgery, and tear substitutes.

B. Lagophthalmos

Lagophthalmos (hare eye, **B**) is the name for incomplete lid closure with infrequent blinking. Besides mechanical causes (cicatricial shortening of the lids, exophthalmos) or unconsciousness, lagophthalmos is usually due to paralysis of the orbicularis oculi muscle in peripheral facial nerve paresis. Because of bilateral cortical innervation, the orbicularis oculi is not affected in supranuclear facial paresis. Three-quarters of cases of peripheral paresis are idiopathic. Peripheral facial nerve lesions are also found with inflammation, petrous temporal fractures, and tumors. **Exposure keratitis** can occur depending on the degree of **Bell's phenomenon**, the physiological upward movement of the eyeball with attempted eyelid closure. Paralytic ectropion, which is usually mild, may also be present. Therapeutically, tear substitutes and bandage contact lenses may be used, and temporary or permanent tarsorrhaphy and canthus repair are performed in severe cases.

C. Blepharospasm

Blepharospasm is characterized by involuntary bilateral contraction of the orbicularis oculi muscle, which is innervated by the facial nerve (**C**). Together with photophobia and epiphora, blepharospasm forms part of the defensive triad in inflammation and superficial injuries of the anterior part of the eye. **Idiopathic (essential) blepharospasm** affects mainly women in middle age. The treatment consists of a combination of medication and psychotherapeutic treatment. **Botulinum toxin** and anticholinergics are successful temporarily. Other causes are degenerative, hereditary, metabolic, vascular and inflammatory brain diseases along with neuroleptic and dopaminergic drugs.

A. Malformations and Anomalies

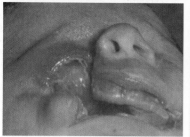

a Complex facial deformity

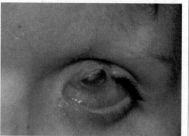

b Complex eye deformity

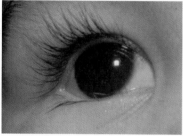

c Epiblepharon

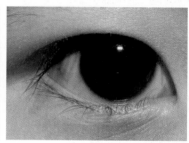

d Epicanthus

B. Lagophthalmos

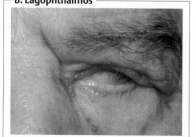

Lagophthalmos in facial nerve paresis

C. Blepharospasm

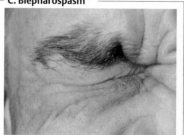

A. Entropion

Entropion means the turning inward of the lid, usually the lower lid. Etiology/pathogenesis. The following are distinguished according to the pathogenesis:

- *Senile entropion* (**Ab, c**) due to slackness of the preseptal part of the orbicularis oculi and of the lid retractors in old age
- *Cicatricial entropion* due to scar contraction of the conjunctiva after burns, corrosive injury, inflammation (especially ocular pemphigoid, Stevens-Johnson syndrome, trachoma), trauma, or surgery
- *Congenital entropion* due to hypertrophy of the marginal zone of the orbicularis oculi
- *Spastic entropion* in blepharospasm, often present as an additional spastic element in senile entropion

Epidemiology. The commonest form by far is senile entropion. There is no sex predisposition.

Clinical features. The clinical appearance is largely determined by the resulting **trichiasis**, the rubbing of the lashes on the cornea and conjunctiva with epiphora and a foreign-body sensation. When chronic, this can lead to severe corneal complications.

Diagnosis. The diagnosis is made clinically.

Differential diagnosis. Epiblepharon must be distinguished in the case of congenital entropion.

Treatment. The symptomatic treatment of trichiasis is by means of (electro-)epilation, cryocoagulation or laser coagulation, or surgical excision. The treatment of choice of entropion is surgical correction by means of Snellen sutures, horizontal shortening of the lid, orbicularis excision, and/or attachment of the lower lid aponeurosis. Marked cicatricial entropion can necessitate replacement of the scarred conjunctival tissue by mucosal grafts. Plaster bandages and tear substitutes are used temporarily.

Prognosis. The prognosis after surgery is good, though the various procedures demonstrate different recurrence rates. Ectropion can result from overcorrection.

B. Ectropion

Ectropion means the turning outward of the lid, usually the lower lid.

Etiology/pathogenesis. The following are distinguished according to the pathogenesis:

- *Senile ectropion* (**Ba, c**) due to slackness of the pretarsal parts of the orbicularis oculi and of the palpebral ligament in old age
- *Cicatricial ectropion* (**Bb**) due to scarring and contraction of the skin and subcutaneous fat after tumors, trauma, burns, and surgery
- *Congenital ectropion* due to hypotrophy of the orbicularis oculi
- *Spastic ectropion* in blepharospasm
- *Paralytic ectropion* due to weakness of the orbicularis oculi in facial nerve paresis

Epidemiology. Senile ectropion is the commonest form. There is no sex predisposition. Paralytic ectropion is apparent in nearly every case of facial nerve paresis but is only mild in expression unless associated with another form.

Clinical features. Epiphora and conjunctivitis are the predominant symptoms. When chronic, conjunctival hypertrophy and keratinization also occur.

Diagnosis. The diagnosis is made clinically.

Differential diagnosis. None.

Treatment. Treatment is surgical by means of cauterization, medial conjunctival repair, or horizontal lid shortening (Bick, Fox, or Kuhnt-Szymanowski method) and in cicatricial ectropion also by Z-plasty, advancement flaps, and free skin grafts. Tear substitutes and Plexiglas shields are also employed.

Prognosis. The prognosis after surgical intervention is good. Entropion can result from overcorrection. Treatment of paralytic ectropion is problematic because of the accompanying **lagophthalmos**.

A. Entropion

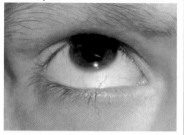

a Upper lid entropion

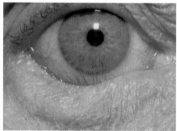

b Senile entropion

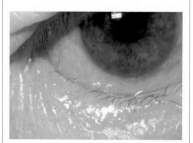

c Senile entropion

B. Ectropion

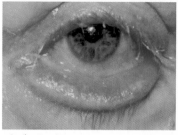

a Senile ectropion

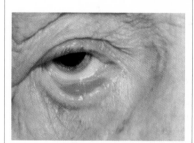

b Cicatricial ectropion

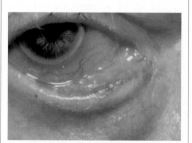

c Senile ectropion, predominantly nasal

A. Ptosis

Ptosis is the term for pathological drooping of the upper lid.

Etiology/pathogenesis. Ptosis can be caused by one or more of the following factors:

- Neurogenic disorders such as congenital or acquired oculomotor paresis (**Aa**), Horner syndrome, Marcus-Gunn phenomenon, or aberrant innervation of the oculomotor nerve
- Congenital or acquired myogenic disorders such as myasthenia gravis, myotonic dystrophy, ocular myopathy, or oculopharyngeal muscular dystrophy
- Levator palpebrae muscle aponeurosis slackness or dehiscence as in senile ptosis (**Ab**) or postoperative ptosis
- Mechanical disorders due to excessive weight of the upper lid (tumors) or scarring of the conjunctiva

Epidemiology. Ptosis is a relatively common finding. The most important causes are acquired oculomotor paresis, Horner syndrome and myasthenia gravis. There is no age or sex predisposition in oculomotor paresis and Horner syndrome. Myasthenia gravis typically affects women in middle age.

Clinical features. Clinically the drooping of one or both upper lids predominates. Depending on the pathogenesis and degree of severity, the patients complain of other symptoms (e.g., restrictions of the visual field) or diminished vision.

In paralysis of the oculomotor nerve, ptosis occurs because of the loss of the levator palpebrae muscle (**paralytic ptosis**). Disorders of eye movement with diplopia (external ophthalmoplegia) and paresis of the sphincter pupillae and ciliary muscle with fixed pupils and accommodation disorders (internal ophthalmoplegia) can be present also. Diabetes mellitus is one of the commonest causes of peripheral lesions of the third cranial nerve. Recurrent ischaemic lesions with acute unilateral and sometimes painful paresis of the extrinsic eye muscles innervated by the oculomotor nerve are characteristic. Nuclear oculomotor lesions are usually associated with slight bilateral ptosis as both levator palpebrae muscles are innervated by a single nuclear region.

In **Horner syndrome** there is a classical triad consisting of ptosis, miosis, and (pseudo-) enophthalmos. Since only the circular fibers of the ciliary muscle are affected in this ocular sympathetic paresis and the function of the levator palpebrae, which is innervated by the oculomotor nerve, is not affected, the unilateral ptosis is often slight.

In the **Marcus-Gunn phenomenon** (**Ac–f**), congenital anomalous innervation leads to elevation of the ptotic lid during masticatory movements and on mouth opening. Simple congenital ptosis is the result of dominantly or recessively inherited dystrophy of the levator palpebrae muscle, which is usually unilateral. It is characterized by defective contraction and relaxation of the muscle. Weakness of the superior rectus muscle is also seen occasionally.

Myasthenia gravis pseudoparalytica is an autoimmune disease and is due to a disorder of neuromuscular stimulus transmission as a result of blocking of the acetylcholine receptors of the motor endplate by circulating polyclonal autoantibodies. There is an increased incidence of other autoimmune diseases. Ocular symptoms (ptosis, diplopia) occur most frequently, followed by speech, chewing, and swallowing disorders. The muscle weakness also affects facial expression (myopathic facies). Three-quarters of patients with myasthenia have eye involvement. Purely ocular myasthenia is present in 20% of cases. The disease is manifested more often after psychological stress and worsens during the course of the day and with fatigue. The usually bilateral, asymmetrical ptosis increases on prolonged upgaze (Simpson test). The muscle weakness improves following injection of an acetylcholinesterase inhibitor (Tensilon or prostigmine test). In 90% of patients with generalized myasthenia and in 50% with purely ocular myasthenia, autoantibodies to acetylcholine receptors can be found in the serum. There is an increased incidence of persistent thymus, thymus hyperplasia, or thymoma.

A. Ptosis

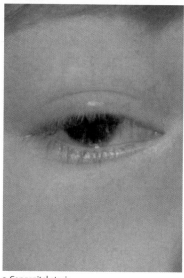

a Congenital ptosis

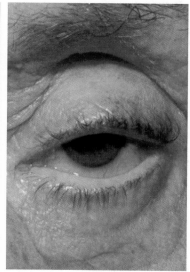

b Senile ptosis

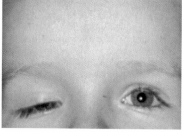

c Marcus–Gunn phenomenon

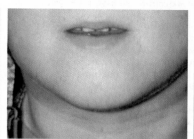

d Marcus–Gunn phenomenon

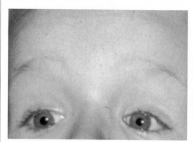

e Marcus–Gunn phenomenon

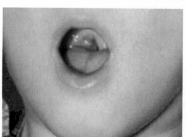

f Marcus–Gunn phenomenon

A. Ptosis (continued)

Myotonic dystrophy (Curschmann-Batten-Steinert syndrome) is an autosomal dominant inherited myopathy with circumscribed muscle dystrophy, myotonic reaction, and various concomitant symptoms such as cataract and gonadal atrophy. Apart from bilateral ptosis, amimia, and atrophy of the temporal muscles (myopathic facies), there is weakness particularly of the sternocleidomastoid, brachioradialis, and fibular muscles.

Ocular myopathy (chronic progressive external ophthalmoplegia) is characterized by progressive ptosis with progressive ocular muscle paresis due to atrophy of the motor nuclear region. As the muscle involvement is strictly symmetrical, double vision is not found even in the advanced stage. In the Kearns-Sayre syndrome (ophthalmoplegia plus), as well as ocular myopathy, tapetoretinal degeneration, cardiac conduction disorders, small stature, and neurological manifestations are also found.

In the autosomal dominant inherited **oculopharyngeal muscular dystrophy** there is paresis of pharyngeal muscles and of the temporalis muscle along with paralysis of the extrinsic ocular muscles.

Diagnosis. The diagnosis of ptosis is made clinically. The Tensilon test (see p. 18) is used to distinguish it from myasthenia gravis.

Differential diagnosis. Pseudoptosis due to an excessively small eyeball (microphthalmos, phthisis bulbi) or contralateral lid retraction, blepharochalasis, or dermatochalasis.

Treatment. The treatment of ptosis depends on the etiology. Congenital or myogenic ptosis can usually be improved by transdermal or transconjunctival levator resection/folding if some residual levator function is preserved. If there is no or only slight levator function, suturing of the tarsus to the frontalis muscle by means of a loop usually produces better results. Tarsoconjunctival resection or reinforcement of the aponeurosis is also employed. Thymectomy demonstrates good results in the treatment of myasthenia gravis. Long-term immunosuppressant treatment with azathioprine and corticosteroids is recommended. Symptomatic treatment with an acetylcholinesterase inhibitor (pyridostigmine) usually shows a rapid improvement in the symptoms but is not suitable for long-term treatment because of diminishing efficacy.

Prognosis. The course and prognosis differ depending on the etiology. While there is no change in Horner syndrome and in most forms of oculomotor paresis, the prognosis is good in diabetic oculomotor paresis with regression within three months. Recurrences are possible. Myasthenia gravis has a chronic progressive course.

B. Blepharochalasis

Bilateral blepharochalasis is caused by acute lid edema. Thinning and atrophy of the skin and stretching and separation of the aponeurosis lead to ptosis (**Ba** and **b**). The function of the levator palpebrae is usually normal and the degree of ptosis is variable. Blepharochalasis is apparent before the age of 20 years in 60%, and women are affected more often. Dominant inheritance has been described. Treatment is surgical.

C. Dermatochalasis

Dermatochalasis is characterized by folds of excessive skin in the upper lid (**Ca** and **b**). If the orbital septum is weakened, this can be associated with a prolapse of the orbital fat. The lid crease is obliterated. Dermatochalasis occurs predominantly at a more advanced age. Patients complain of a heavy sensation in the region of the eyes and in severe cases of visual impairment. Treatment is surgical by an upper lid lift with excision of the excess skin.

B. Blepharochalasis

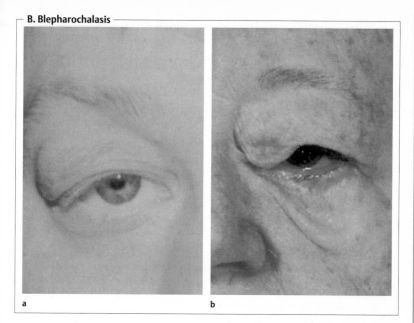

a   b

C. Dermatochalasis

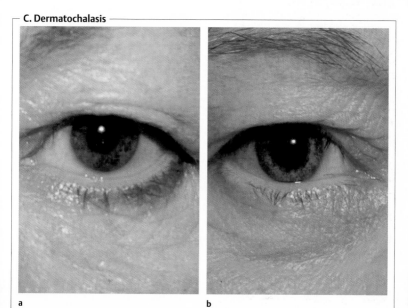

a   b

A. Inflammation of the Lid Margin (Marginal Blepharitis)

Marginal blepharitis (**Aa** and **b**) is a chronic inflammation of the lid margin. It is often accompanied by secondary changes in the conjunctiva and cornea.

Etiology/pathogenesis. Staphylococcal infections and seborrhea are the most important pathogenic factors. In addition, instability of the tear film is nearly always found.

Epidemiology. This is the commonest disorder of the outer eye. Marginal blepharitis often begins in childhood and women are affected more frequently.

Clinical features. The patients complain of chronic irritation of the eyes with burning and itching. Mixed forms of staphylococcal (ulcerative blepharitis) and seborrheic (squamous blepharitis) inflammation are typical. The staphylococcal form is due to chronic infection of the lash follicles by staphylococci. As well as dilated blood vessels (rosettes), encrusted scales are found at the base of the lashes. Trichiasis, loss (madarosis), or depigmentation (poliosis) of the lashes can also occur. Scarring of the lid margin (entropion, ectropion) or secondary conjunctival and corneal inflammation can occur in the late stage. Seborrheic blepharitis is the result of overproduction by the meibomian and Zeis glands. The excess free fatty acids lead to irritation of the lid margin, conjunctiva, and cornea. Other seborrheic skin changes are frequently found. The lid margins demonstrate a typical waxy sheen. The lashes are greasy and stuck together. Soft greasy scales are found over the entire lid margin. Small drops of oil are visible along the openings of the ducts of the meibomian glands.

Diagnosis. The diagnosis is made clinically.

Differential diagnosis. Rosacea and other dermatoses involving the lids.

Treatment. Lid hygiene is in the foreground of treatment. Warm compresses and artificial tears often relieve the symptoms. Antibiotic eyedrops are additionally used in staphylococcal blepharitis. Severe secondary complications occasionally necessitate the use of corticosteroids.

Prognosis. This is a chronic disorder the treatment of which is often unsatisfactory and which usually cannot be cured. Secondary changes are less severe in the seborrheic form than in staphylococcal blepharitis.

B. Allergic Inflammation of the Lid (Allergic Dermatitis)

Despite the usually multifactorial pathogenesis, lid dermatitis and eczema (**Ba** and **b**) are usually classified according to the main pathogenesis. Most lid dermatitis and eczema are allergic in origin. **Contact allergies of the delayed type** are most common, followed by atopic and irritant eczema. Most patients are women, and the average age of affected patients is 45 years. Apart from cosmetics, ophthalmological preparations and contact lens care products often have allergenic or irritant effects. Erythema, severe itching, and also scaling in the later stages are typical clinical signs. Confirmation of contact sensitization is done by skin testing. Apart from avoidance of the allergen, mast cell stabilizers and antihistamines are used in treatment, with corticosteroids and cyclosporin A (ciclosporin) in severe and chronic cases. Besides the lichenification of the skin of the lid, typical stigmata of atopy are often found in **atopic dermatitis**, such as a double Dennie-Morgan crease in the lower lid, loss of the lateral part of the eyebrows (Hertoghe's sign), and haloing of the eyes. The lid eczema may be the only manifestation of atopy. Secondary contact allergy can also be detected in about one-third of patients. Marginal blepharitis with marked instability of the tear film is frequently found as a complication. Herpetic blepharoconjunctivitis is a rare complication.

A. Marginal Blepharitis

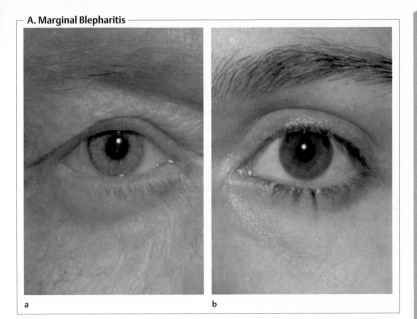

a   b

B. Allergic Dermatitis

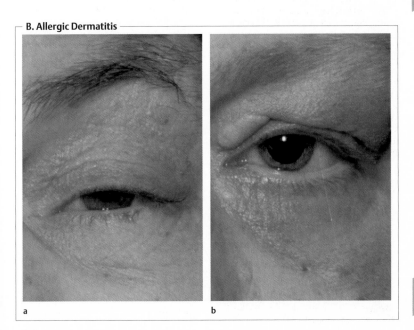

a   b

A. Infectious Inflammation of the Lid

In local infection following trauma, insect bites, hematoma, or spread from purulent sinusitis or osteomyelitis, severe erythema and swelling of the lid (pseudoptosis) with fever and the development of a **lid abscess** (**Aa**) or **lid cellulitis** (**Ab**) can occur with the risk of intracerebral extension. Typical pathogens are staphylococci and streptococci, rarely anaerobic bacteria. Mixed infections are frequent. Apart from establishing the cause, the treatment consists of giving high-dose broad-spectrum antibiotics. If resolution or spontaneous perforation do not occur, incision, irrigation, and drainage is performed. In contrast to orbital cellulitis, eye movements are always intact.

Lid erysipelas occurs rarely. Together with severe pain and usually a high fever, a sharply demarcated intense erythema develops that does not necessarily have the typical tongues-of-flame shape in the lid. The cause is a wound infection with (-hemolytic streptococci. High-dose antibiotic therapy is necessary to prevent extension. Involvement of the lids in syphilis, anthrax, tuberculosis, leprosy, and diphtheria has also been described rarely.

Lid herpes is an infection of the skin of the lid with the herpes simplex virus (**Ac**). This is usually due to reactivation of latent infection, more rarely to primary infection. After lessening of maternal antibody protection, the first infection often occurs in early childhood due to direct contact or droplet infection from herpetic lesions from healthy chronic shedders. Only 1 % of the initial infections are clinically apparent, usually as herpetic gingivostomatitis. The neurotropic viruses persist in the body even after the inflammation has subsided. Recurrences occur through irritation of latently infected neurons after febrile infections, sun exposure, menstruation, trauma, and gastrointestinal disorders, and also due to immunosuppressant, hormonal, and psychological factors. There is severe itching and a sensation of tension; the typical cluster of vesicles develops on a reddened background and heals without scarring after 8–10 days. Regional lymph node swelling is possible. Besides the lips and genitals, the skin of the face, particularly the lid, is typically affected. Involvement of the conjunctiva and cornea is not infrequent. Treatment is symptomatic. Antiviral ointments hasten healing.

Ophthalmic zoster (shingles), when it affects the face, is an infection of the gasserian ganglion and the area innervated by the ophthalmic nerve (V_1) by the varicella zoster virus (**Ad**). The disease is an expression of a reinfection or more often activation of the neurotropic viruses even years after the primary infection. Severe neuralgiform pain occurs initially. Skin erythema develops with initially clear tense vesicles, the content of which leaves behind yellowish dried and brownish crusts and scars. The disease is of great importance because of the potentially serious ophthalmological complications. Treatment consists of local and systemic administration of virostatic drugs.

Under conditions of poor hygiene **crab lice** (*Phthirus pubis*) or more rarely **head lice** (*Pediculus humanus capitis*) can infest the lid margin. They are spread by direct contact. The lice lodge on the lid margin between the cilia and lay their nits on the shafts of the eyelashes, where they have the appearance of small black grains. The patients complain of severe itching. Marginal blepharitis is often found. Treatment consists of removal of the lice and nits and administration of topical parasympathomimetics.

Ticks (**Ae**) can also occasionally infest the lid margin. They are removed completely with tweezers. Transmission of borreliosis or early summer meningoencephalitis is also possible on the lid.

A. Infectious Inflammations of the Lid

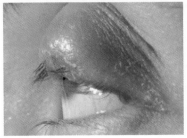

a Lid abscess

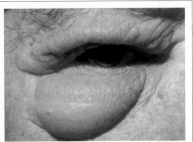

b Lid phlegmon

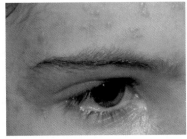

c Herpes simplex

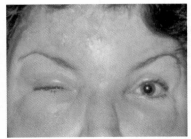

d Herpes zoster

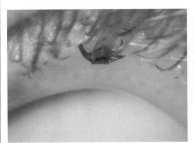

e Tick in the upper row of lashes

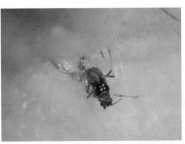

f Fly larva in the lower row of lashes

A. Hordeolum

A stye (external hordeolum, **A**) is an acute inflammation of the Zeis or Moll glands with pain and swelling. Similarly painful inflammation of the meibomian glands is called an internal hordeolum.

Etiology/pathogenesis. The cause is folliculitis or an abscess in the Zeis or Moll glands located superficially at the roots of the lashes, or a staphylococcal infection of the meibomian glands located in the tarsus.

Epidemiology. There is no age or sex predisposition.

Clinical features. There is localized inflamed swelling of the lid margin. Several hordeola are often found adjacent to one another. There can be general malaise. Swelling of preauricular lymph nodes and fever are also frequent. Lid abscess and orbital cellulitis are rare.

Diagnosis. The diagnosis is made clinically. Diabetes mellitus must be excluded if there is repeated occurrence.

Differential diagnosis. Marginal blepharitis, chalazion.

Treatment. Dry heat infrared warming, and local disinfectant and antibiotic therapy hasten coalescence. Lancing may become necessary if spontaneous healing does not occur.

Prognosis. Benign, occasionally recurrent.

B. Chalazion

A chalazion (**Ba**) is the result of obstruction of the duct of a meibomian gland, which is usually idiopathic, with secondary lipogranulomatous inflammation (**Bb**).

Epidemiology. There is no age or sex predisposition. There is a higher incidence of chalazion in seborrheic dermatitis, rosacea, and diabetes mellitus.

Clinical features. The appearance is of a pale, round, firm lesion of the lid. With secondary bacterial infection it is difficult to distinguish from an internal hordeolum. Astigmatism with a reduction in vision can be induced by pressure on the eyeball.

Diagnosis. The diagnosis is made clinically.

Differential diagnosis. Hordeolum, pyogenic granuloma (**Bc**), sebaceous gland carcinoma.

Treatment. The cysts can be incised and removed by curetting. Steroid injection can initiate remission.

Prognosis. Benign, occasionally recurrent.

C. Molluscum Contagiosum

The wartlike lesions of molluscum contagiosum (**C**) are usually numerous and consist of virally induced papules with a central indentation.

Etiology/pathogenesis. Molluscum contagiosum is caused by DNA viruses of the poxvirus group. Transmission is by direct contact, autoinoculation, perinatally, and by sexual contact. The incubation period varies between 1 week and 6 months.

Epidemiology. The incidence of molluscum contagiosum is increased in children and immunosuppressed patients. There is no sex predisposition.

Clinical features. There are usually numerous skin-colored papules ranging in size from a pinhead to pea-sized with an indented center. With pressure, a cheesy contagious material is expressed. Concomitant conjunctivitis is often observed when the lesions are near the lid margin.

Diagnosis. The diagnosis is made clinically.

Differential diagnosis. Common wart, milium, keratoacanthoma, granuloma, chalazion, basal cell carcinoma.

Treatment. Molluscum contagiosum lesions are incised and removed by curetting or excision.

Prognosis. Benign, recurrent. Spontaneous remissions are possible even after years.

D. Common Warts

Common warts are occasionally found on the lid (**D**). These pea-sized, hemispherical hard nodules with a prickly surface are the result of infection with a papilloma virus. The incubation period is 6 weeks to 20 months. They sometimes occur in groups as filiform warts. The therapeutic options available include removal with a curette, cryotherapy, and electrocoagulation.

A. Hordeolum

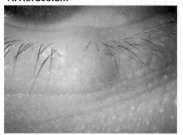

B. Chalazion

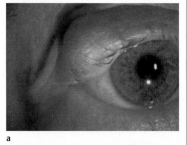

a

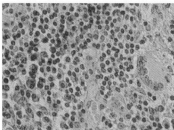

b Histological section, ca. 40: lymphocytes, epithelioid cells, and foreign-body giant cells

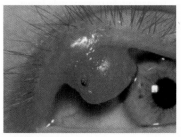

c Pyogenic granuloma

C. Molluscum Contagiosum

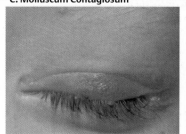

D. Common Wart

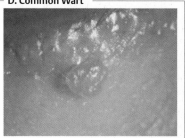

A. Dermoid cyst

The dermoid cyst (**A**) is a benign mature teratoma.

Etiology/pathogenesis. The cyst is a congenital lesion due to deep sequestration of epidermal tissue.

Epidemiology. Manifestation extends from birth to early adulthood. There is no sex predisposition.

Clinical features. An bulging elastic tumor, ca. 1 cm, of variable mobility usually develops in the upper temporal lid region. An intraorbital location is possible.

Diagnosis. The diagnosis is made clinically.

Differential diagnosis. Tumors of the lacrimal gland, mucocele, hemangioma, lymphangioma, inflammatory processes.

Treatment. Surgical excision is the treatment of choice. Observation is also possible depending on the size.

Prognosis. Benign, not recurrent, no known risk of malignant transformation.

B. Capillary Hemangioma

The capillary hemangioma (**B**) is a benign neoplasm of blood vessels.

Etiology/pathogenesis. Unknown.

Epidemiology. There is a greater incidence in females.

Clinical features. A usually superficial bright red to purple lesion is observed usually on the surface of the upper lid ca. 1 cm in size and of spongy consistency.

Diagnosis. The diagnosis is made clinically.

Differential diagnosis. Cavernous hemangioma, nevus flammeus, lymphangioma.

Treatment. Steroid induction of spontaneous regression along with laser and cryocoagulation are possible.

Prognosis. Benign, not recurrent. Regression with complete remission in up to 90 % in the first years of life.

C. Xanthelasma

Xanthelasmas (**C**) are flat yellowish tumors in the region of the medial canthus, which are due to deposits of cholesterol in macrophages.

Etiology/pathogenesis. Approximately 50 % of affected patients suffer from hypercholesterolemia, otherwise it is due to a local disorder of lipid metabolism.

Epidemiology. The disease affects older women more often.

Clinical features. Bilateral, yellowish, flat plaques are most commonly found at the medial canthus.

Diagnosis. The diagnosis is made clinically.

Differential diagnosis. None.

Treatment. Apart from treatment of the underlying disease, the main treatments are surgical excision or laser ablation for cosmetic reasons.

Prognosis. Benign, recurrent.

D. Keratoacanthoma

The keratoacanthoma (**D**) is a spherical epithelial tumor.

Etiology/pathogenesis. Unknown.

Epidemiology. The tumor occurs predominantly in later life. There is no sex predisposition.

Clinical features. Within a few weeks, a broad-based tumor 0.5–1 cm in diameter with a central keratinous crater develops, which resolves after a few weeks leaving a flat scar.

Diagnosis. The diagnosis is made clinically.

Differential diagnosis. Squamous cell carcinoma, basal cell carcinoma, common wart, actinic keratosis.

Treatment. Because it is sometimes difficult to distinguish it from squamous cell carcinoma, surgical excision with histological examination is recommended.

Prognosis. Benign, not recurrent, no known risk of malignant transformation.

E. Other

In addition to the described tumors, benign lesions of the lid also include seborrheic and actinic keratoses, **nevi** (**Ea**), congenital hemangiomas, lymphangiomas, fibromas and neurofibromas, along with epidermoid cysts. The **cutaneous horn** (**Eb**) occupies a particular position. This is a yellow-brown growth of the skin of various histogenesis, which is excised because of the risk of malignant transformation.

A. Dermoid Cyst

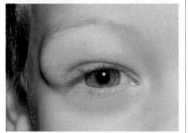

B. Capillary Hemangioma

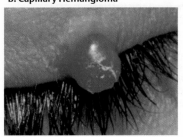

C. Xanthelasma

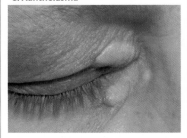

D. Keratoacanthoma

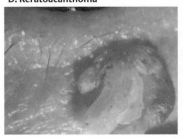

E. Other

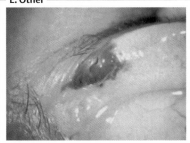

a Nevus

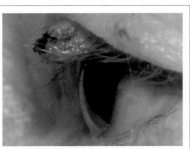

b Cutaneous horn

A. Basal Cell Carcinoma

The basal cell carcinoma is a semimalignant skin tumor derived from the epidermal basal cells and the cells of the outer hair follicle sheaths.

Etiology/pathogenesis. The etiology has not been finally elucidated. Chronic light exposure is important. Precancerous forms are unknown.

Epidemiology. The tumor occurs typically in later life and accounts for 90% of malignant and 20% of all lid tumors. There is no sex predisposition.

Clinical features. Different forms are distinguished according to the growth behavior:

- Nodular (solid) type (**Aa**): 75%; slow-growing nontender nodule, central ulceration (**Ab**), pearly shimmer, telangiectasias
- Pigmented type (**Ac**): 10%
- Sclerosing (morphea) type (**Ad**)
- Superficial type

Mixed forms are frequent. The preferred location is the medial lower lid. The tumor growth is infiltrating and destructive.

Diagnosis. The diagnosis is made clinically and histologically.

Differential diagnosis. Other malignant tumors of the lid, keratoacanthoma, seborrheic keratosis, common wart.

Treatment. Surgical excision followed by plastic reconstruction is the treatment of choice. Cryotherapy and radiotherapy are also used occasionally with good results. Prognosis. Recurrence occurs in 5–15%. Metastasis occurs in 0.1%.

B. Squamous Cell Carcinoma

Squamous cell carcinoma (**B**) is a rapidly growing and metastasizing tumor of epithelial origin.

Etiology/pathogenesis. The etiology has not been finally elucidated. There is a predisposition with light exposure. Development from precancerous lesions and de novo is known to occur.

Epidemiology. There is a higher incidence in the male sex and in later life. The tumor accounts for nearly 10% of lid malignancies and 2% of all lid tumors.

Clinical features. Over months, a flat erythematous lesion with crusts and ulceration develops, which later becomes nodular, papillomatous, or cystic.

Diagnosis. The diagnosis is made clinically and histologically.

Differential diagnosis. Keratoacanthoma, other malignant tumors and precancerous lesions of the lid.

Treatment. The treatment of choice is histologically confirmed excision. Prognosis. Recurrence occurs in 10–20%. Metastasis occurs in 1–21%. Mortality is 10–15%.

C. Sebaceous Cyst Carcinoma

Sebaceous cyst carcinomas (**C**) are rapidly growing and metastasizing tumors that originate predominantly from meibomian and Zeis glands.

Etiology/pathogenesis. The etiology is unknown.

Epidemiology. Sebaceous cyst carcinomas occur mainly in later life. Women appear to be affected slightly more often. The tumor accounts for 0.2–0.7% of all and about 1% of malignant lid tumors.

Clinical features. The tumor, which is located predominantly in the upper lid, commences as a firm nonpainful tumor, similar to a chalazion. Late ulceration is possible. There is often a loss of eyelashes.

Diagnosis. The diagnosis is made clinically and histologically.

Differential diagnosis. Chalazion, other malignant tumors and precancerous lesions of the lid. Treatment. Mainly surgical excision.

Prognosis. Recurrence occurs in 10–40% and lymphogenous metastasis in 17–28%. The mortality is 5–15%.

Other, rare malignant tumors of the lid include malignant melanoma, Merkel cell carcinoma, Kaposi sarcoma, chondrosarcoma, and metastases.

A. Basal Cell Carcinoma

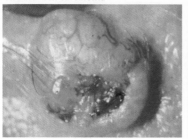

a Nodular type

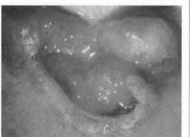

b Basal cell carcinoma, severely ulcerating

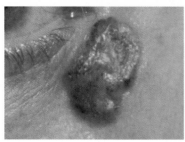

c Pigmented type

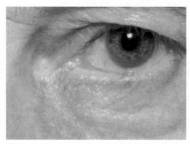

d Morphea type: medial lower lid and inner canthus

B. Squamous Cell Carcinoma

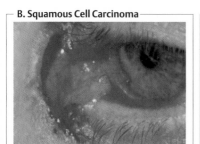

C. Sebaceous Cyst Carcinoma

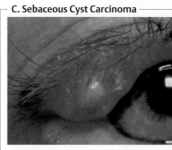

A. Surgical Alterations

A frequent unwanted consequence of surgery is the development of a **scar keloid**. This is a tough, flat or stringy, sometimes itchy proliferation of connective tissue, which develops depending on individual and ethnic predisposition weeks to months after the procedure in the region of the operation scar. In contrast to **hypertrophic scars**, extension is possible even to originally undamaged skin. The treatment consists of intralesional injection of corticosteroids, radiotherapy, a pressure bandage, and possibly surgical revision in the case of scar contractures. In the course of postoperative wound healing, **lid deformities** can occur, which sometimes necessitate revision operations. These include mainly ectropion, entropion, and ptosis.

B. Trauma

Lid trauma is a frequent injury. Approximately 75% of the patients are male. The average age is between 30 and 60 years. Over half of the injuries are due to blunt trauma due to falls, acts of violence (**Ba**), road traffic accidents, and work and sports injuries (**Bb**). In addition to lacerations and bites (**Bc–e**), corrosive injuries and burns (**Bf**) are also frequent. In about half of all lid injuries there is also injury of the globe, which can extend from superficial injury to severe eyeball penetration and rupture. Severe, extensive and multiple lacerations of the facial region after road traffic accidents have become rare as a result of seatbelt laws in cars and the introduction of shatter-proof glass. Lid injuries are often found in conjunction with extensive head and facial injuries. Because of the collateral circulation and the loose structure of the lid connective tissue, hemorrhage and lid edema develop rapidly, which can often spread to the uninjured side. Fractures of the orbit, midface, and base of the skull should be excluded. Depending on the depth and extent of the lid injury, abrasions, contusions, lacerations, avulsions, and puncture wounds are distinguished. With full-thickness defects of the upper lid, the levator palpebrae muscle is often involved, which can lead to posttraumatic ptosis. With lid injuries in the medial canthus, there are often injuries of the lacrimal ducts. In particular, because of the divided insertion of the medial palpebral ligament, careful repair of this area is important to prevent posttraumatic lid deformities. The risk of infection after lid injuries can be regarded as low. In the treatment of lid trauma, a distinction is made between primary management and repair, which may be required later. The goal of the primary treatment is restoration of the anatomy and normal function. Management of the lid injury depends on the degree of the damage and extends from simple interrupted sutures and suture of the lid margins to large advancement flaps. Deformities of the lids can occur in the course of wound healing due to scar formation, necessitating further revision operations. The commonest posttraumatic deformities are ectropion, entropion with trichiasis, deformity of the canthus, and ptosis.

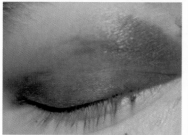

a Lid hematoma due to a blow from a fist

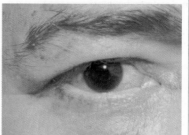

b Lid hematoma due to impact of a squash ball

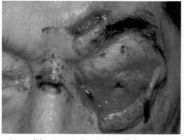

c Severe lid trauma with avulsion of lid margin and loss of tissue

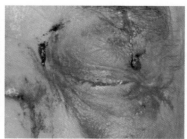

d Multiple lacerations (windshield injury))

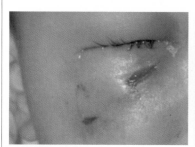

e Dog bite injury

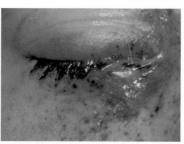

f Explosive injury

A. Congenital Anomalies of the Lacrimal Gland

Complete absence of the lacrimal gland (**aplasia**), displacement (**ectopia**), lacrimal gland cysts (**dacryops, A**), or lacrimal gland fistulas are rare.

B. Dry Eye: Sicca Syndrome

Complex qualitative and quantitative disorders of the production and surface adhesion of the tear film.

Etiology/pathogenesis. Multifactorial, caused by ophthalmological and general diseases and by exogenous factors (**B, Table 1**).

Epidemiology. Very common. Symptoms in ca. 22 % of women and 10 % of men between 55 and 60 years. Signs of keratoconjunctivitis sicca in 20 % of women and 15 % of men between 45 and 54 years.

Clinical features. Dryness, sensation of pressure, pain, burning, scratching, foreign-body sensation, photophobia, lid swelling, corneal edema, corneal epithelial filaments, conjunctival folds parallel to the lid margins (LIPCOF), tear meniscus irregular and/or reduced < 0.2 mm.

Diagnosis. The diagnosis is made clinically and by means of tests, including the Schirmer test < 10 mm/5 min, Jones basal secretion test < 10 mm/5 min, break-up time < 10 s.

Differential diagnosis. Infection, asthenopia.

Treatment. Tear substitute, moisture chamber, glasses with side protection, punctum plug.

Treatment of the underlying disease. Reduction in exogenous factors (smoke, dust, night work, etc.).

Prognosis. Rarely major symptoms. Increased bacterial superinfection.

C. Acute Dacryoadenitis

Sudden unilateral tender swelling of the lacrimal gland.

Etiology/pathogenesis. See **C, Table 2**.

Epidemiology. Usually middle-aged women.

Clinical features. Erythema, swelling, tenderness of the lateral third of the upper lid (**S-shaped curve of the upper lid, C**), conjunctival chemosis, palpable preauricular lymph nodes, fever, general malaise, leukocytosis.

Diagnosis. The diagnosis is made clinically.

Differential diagnosis. Lid/orbital cellulitis, hordeolum, lid abscess, sinusitis, erysipelas.

Treatment. Antibiotic therapy. Incision and drainage.

Prognosis. The disease lasts 8–10 days.

D. Chronic Dacryoadenitis

Painless, slightly inflammatory swelling of the lacrimal gland, unilateral or bilateral.

Etiology/pathogenesis. Sequela of acute dacryoadenitis, granulomatous diseases (**D, Table 3**).

Epidemiology. Usually men over 40 years.

Clinical features. Painless swelling of the lateral upper lid.

Diagnosis. The diagnosis is made clinically. Further investigations depending on the underlying disease. Biopsy.

Differential diagnosis. Tumor, dermoid, osteomyelitis, systemic diseases.

Treatment. Treatment of the underlying disease.

Prognosis. Depending on the underlying disease.

E. Pleomorphic Adenoma (Benign Mixed-Cell Tumor)

Etiology/pathogenesis. Unknown. Benign tumor of epithelial and myoepithelial cells.

Epidemiology. Commonest epithelial tumor of the lacrimal gland (50 %). Age peak at 4th–5th decade. The ratio of men to women is 1.5 : 1 to 2 : 1.

Clinical features. Painless, slowly growing tumor. Visual changes and double vision are not reported. Displacement of the eyeball downward and nasally.

Diagnosis. CT shows a sharply demarcated tumor. Bone atrophy possible. On MRI the tumor appears hypointense on T1-weighted imaging and hyperintense on T2-weighted imaging. Eyeball deformation is possible.

Differential diagnosis. Adenoid cystic carcinoma.

Treatment. Complete excision including the pseudocapsule. Incisional biopsy leads to a high rate of recurrence.

Prognosis. Five-year survival rate of 99 %. Recurrences possible after incomplete excision, malignant transformation also possible.

A. Congenital Abnormalities of the Lacrimal Gland

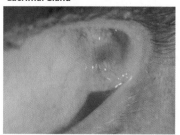

Lacrimal gland cyst

C. Acute Dacryoadenitis

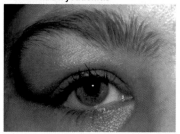

S-shaped curve of the upper lid

Table 2 Etiology/pathogenesis of acute dacryoadenitis

• Bacterial	• Viral
– Staphylococci	– Mumps
– Streptococci	– Measles
– Gonococci	– Scarlet fever
	– Mononucleosis
	– Herpes zoster

B. Sicca Syndrome

Table 1 Causes of sicca syndrome

- General diseases
  - Diabetes mellitus
  - Thyroid diseases: hypothyroidism, endocrine ophthalmopathy, Hashimoto thyroiditis
  - Sjögren syndrome, rheumatoid arthritis, SLE (systemic lupus erythematosus), Wegener granulomatosis, scleroderma
  - Skin diseases: neurodermatitis, acne rosacea, allergies
  - Pregnancy

- External influences
  - Smoke, dry heating, air conditioning
  - Night work
  - Contact lenses
  - Cosmetics

- Medications
  - Analgesics
  - Antiarrhythmics
  - Antihistamines
  - Antihypertensives
  - Hormones
  - Lipid-lowering drugs
  - Psychotropic medications
  - Synthetic retinoids
  - Virostatic drugs
  - Cytostatic drugs

- Diseases of the eye
  - Systemic, infectious, tumor, or surgical damage to the lacrimal gland
  - Conditions of the conjunctiva: trachoma, pemphigoid, allergies, operations, Stevens–Johnson syndrome, burns, corrosive injury, radiation
  - Conditions of the cornea: dystrophies, previous keratoplasty
  - Lid deformities, lid closure deficit, blepharitis

D. Chronic Dacryocystitis

Table 3 Pathogenesis/pathogenesis of chronic dacryoadenitis

- Unhealed acute dacryoadenitis
- Chronic conjunctivitis
- Tuberculosis
- Syphilis
- Leprosy
- Sarcoidosis
- Actinomycosis
- Nocardiosis
- Trachoma

E. Pleomorphic Adenoma

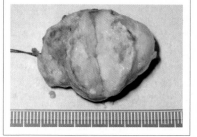

A. Adenoid Cystic Carcinoma

Etiology/pathogenesis. Not known.

Epidemiology. Commonest malignant, second commonest epithelial lacrimal gland tumor (25–30%). Age peak in women about 40 years.

Clinical features. Rapidly growing. Pain with tumor infiltration of nerves or bone.

Diagnosis. On CT, roundish poorly demarcated space-occupying lesion with irregular surface and bone destruction. MRI shows cystic isointense or hyperintense changes in the T1-weighted image.

Differential diagnosis. See **A, Table 1**.

Treatment. Radical resection. Radiotherapy.

Prognosis. Five-year survival rate of 21%. Recurrences and metastasis to the lungs. The prognosis depends on the histological grade.

B. Diseases of the Lacrimal Ducts

The hallmark of all diseases of the lacrimal ducts is **epiphora**. Epiphora immediately post-natally is due to atresia or stenosis of the lacrimal ducts, especially of Hasner's valve. **Signs of inflammation** point to infection, which can be **acute** or **chronic** and appear as **canaliculitis** or **dacryocystitis**. Tumors are a rarer cause of epiphora. Signs suggestive of malignancy are:

- Development of mass above the medial palpebral ligament
- Telangiectasia overlying lacrimal sac swelling
- Bloody secretion, nosebleed, bloody reflux after irrigation of the lacrimal duct

C. Acute Dacryocystitis

Etiology/pathogenesis. Partial or complete obstruction of the nasolacrimal duct with inflammation due to infection, tumor, foreign bodies, after trauma or due to granulomatous diseases.

Epidemiology. Adults between 50 and 60 years.

Clinical features. Epiphora; acute, unilateral, painful inflammation of the lacrimal sac; pus emerging from the lacrimal punctum; fever; general malaise. Pain radiates to the forehead and teeth.

Diagnosis. Diagnosis is made clinically. Swab and culture with antibiotic sensitivity.

Differential diagnosis. Orbital cellulitis, inflammation of the paranasal sinuses, erysipelas.

Treatment. Conservative: see **C, Table 2**. For decompression, freeze the skin (with ethyl chloride), then make the incision. Dacryocystorhinostomy is often necessary later.

Prognosis. Spontaneous discharge of the pus into the ethmoid cells, conjunctival sac, and nose is possible. This can lead to chemosis, lid edema, and erysipelas, more rarely to orbital cellulitis.

D. Chronic Dacryocystitis

Etiology/pathogenesis. Congenital or idiopathic obstructions of the nasolacrimal duct, e.g., due to unhealed acute dacryocystitis, dacryoliths, foreign bodies, tumors, diseases of the surrounding structures (sinusitis, tumors), trauma.

Epidemiology. See acute dacryocystitis.

Clinical features. Epiphora; signs of inflammation are absent; large amounts of mucopurulent secretion drain on pressure over the lacrimal sac.

Diagnosis. Swab and culture, lacrimal duct probing.

Differential diagnosis. None.

Treatment. See **C, Table 2**. Dacryocystorhinostomy.

E. Trauma of the Lacrimal Ducts

These injuries often occur together with lid and facial injuries, particularly with injuries of the nasal canthus. The canaliculi are affected in 70%, more rarely the lacrimal sac (20%) and the nasolacrimal duct (10%). The defect and the canaliculus can be located by thorough inspection under the operating microscope and irrigation with methylene blue or fluorescein. If fractures or foreign bodies are suspected, radiography of the orbit in two planes or CT is indicated. Therapeutically, the earliest possible reconstruction with silastic intubation of the lacrimal ducts should be attempted. The prognosis depends on the extent of the injury. Lid deformities and stenosis of the lacrimal duct system are possible.

A. Adenoid Cystic Carcinoma

Table 1 Differential diagnosis of tumors in the upper temporal quadrant of the orbit

- Benign
  - Dacryops
  - All forms of dacryoadenitis
  - Pleomorphic adenoma
  - Dermoid cyst
  - Benign lymphoid lacrimal gland tumor
  - Eosinophilic granuloma
  - Aneurysmal bone cyst
  - Cholesterol granuloma

- Malignant
  - Adenoid cystic carcinoma
  - Pleomorphic adenocarcinoma
  - Mucoepidermoid carcinoma
  - Squamous epithelial carcinoma
  - Oncocytoma
  - Malignant lymphoma
  - Metastases

B. Diseases of the Lacrimal Ducts

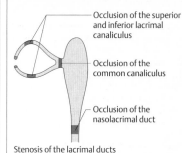

Occlusion of the superior and inferior lacrimal canaliculus

Occlusion of the common canaliculus

Occlusion of the nasolacrimal duct

Stenosis of the lacrimal ducts

D. Chronic Dacryocystitis

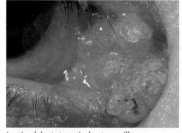

Lacrimal duct stenosis due to papilloma

C. Acute Dacryocystitis

Table 2 Treatment of acute canaliculitis/dacryocystitis

- Bacterial
  - Local: gentamicin eye drops 5 times daily and gentamicin eye ointment at night for 14 days; disinfectant dressings with Rivanol solution 1:1000; xylometazoline eye drops t.i.d. to reduce swelling
  - Systemic: e.g., dicloxacillin p.o. For 10–14 days
  - Actinomycetes: tetracycline eye ointment t.i.d.

- Chlamydia
  - Local: tetracycline, ofloxacin, erythromycin eye ointment t.i.d. for 6 weeks
  - Systemic: tetracycline, erythromycin, doxycycline, or sulfamethoxazole p.o. for 3 weeks

- Fungi
  - E.g., natamycin eye ointment 1–2 hourly

- Viruses
  - *Varicella zoster:* aciclovir 800 mg 5 tabs daily for 7 days, aciclovir eye ointment 5 times daily continued for 3 days after healing

E. Trauma of the Lacrimal Ducts

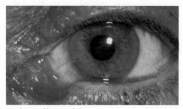

Avulsion of lacrimal duct

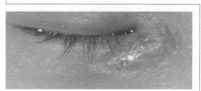

Acute dacryocystitis with persistent Hasner membrane

A. Symptoms of Orbital Diseases

The orbit has close topographical relations to the paranasal sinuses and is linked to the interior of the skull through the optic canal and the superior orbital fissure. Thus, primary orbital processes can extend into the paranasal sinuses and the region of the chiasm, and conversely processes arising primarily in these regions can involve the orbit secondarily. Extension of primary intraocular diseases into the orbit and of primary intraorbital processes into the eyeball is likewise possible.

The pyramid-shaped orbit is bounded anteriorly by the eyeball and the orbital septum and otherwise by bone. The important diseases of the orbit, namely inflammation, tumors and injury-related hemorrhage, are usually associated with an increase in the volume and pressure in the orbit. Orbital symptoms are therefore explained mostly by displacement and/or compression of orbital structures and the eyeball.

The symptoms of orbital diseases are:

- **Exophthalmos** (**Aa–c**), protrusion of the eye (proptosis), is the main symptom of a space-occupying process. Space-occupying lesions located in the muscle funnel (intraconal), such as optic glioma and optic sheath meningioma, lead to protrusion axially and forward. An extraconal increase in volume, in contrast, usually leads to displacement of the eye in the direction opposite to that of the pathological process. As a rule, exophthalmos can be identified when observed from the side. It is measured with a Hertel exophthalmometer, which measures the distance of the anterior pole of the cornea from the lateral margin of the bony orbit, and comparison of the two sides is particularly important. A greatly enlarged eye, e.g., in high myopia or buphthalmos, and also enophthalmos of the opposite side, can mimic exophthalmos ("pseudo-exophthalmos").

- **Enophthalmos** (see p. 47, **Ac**), the sinking backward of the eye, is the sign of volume deficit in the orbit. In old age this is due to atrophy of the orbital fat pad. The cause of unilateral enophthalmos is usually a fracture of the orbital bones (especially the floor of the orbit and ethmoid cells) with displacement of orbital tissue. Processes associated with tissue contraction such as some breast cancer metastases can produce enophthalmos. The enophthalmos in Horner syndrome is usually only slight. The upper lid is often lower in enophthalmos. Enophthalmos is also measured with the Hertel exophthalmometer. A reduction in the size of the eye as in congenital microphthalmos or phthisis bulbi can mimic enophthalmos.

- **A motility deficit (strabismus, Ac)** is caused by the fact that space-occupying and destructive processes in the orbit often reduce the mobility of the eyeball by interfering directly with the ocular muscles (mechanical paresis) or by damaging the motor nerves (neurogenic paresis). If there is a difference in the reduction in eyeball motility between the two sides, strabismus results, usually with double vision.

- **Exposure keratitis** and sometimes a corneal ulcer can develop in exophthalmos as blinking and moistening of the surface of the eye are impaired.

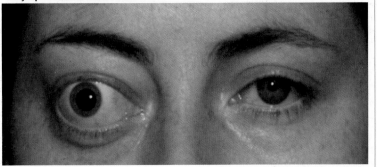

a Exophthalmos on the right with optic glioma; retraction of the upper lid (pupil dilated by medication)

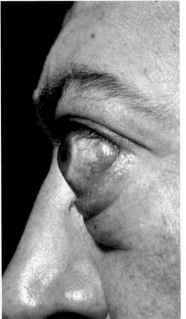

b Exophthalmos seen from the side

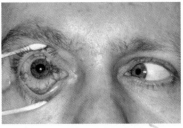

c Inflammatory orbital tumor on the right with exophthalmos and dilated episcleral vessels; massive restriction of eyeball movement on looking to the right

A. Symptoms of Orbital Diseases (continued)

Other symptoms of orbital diseases:

- **Disorders of visual function** can occur when an orbital space-occupying lesion compresses the optic nerve directly or indirectly through an increase in the pressure in the orbit, thus leading to a loss of visual field or visual acuity. Lesions of the optic nerve with loss of visual function also occur not infrequently because of injuries or orbital infections. A reduction in vision also results when there is central corneal opacification due to exposure keratitis.

- Swelling of the head of the optic nerve (**papilledema**) is a frequent though rather non-specific finding in orbital processes. In contrast to papilledema due to raised intracranial pressure, papilledema because of processes in the orbit is often associated early with a reduction in function.

- More prolonged optic nerve compression leads to a loss of ganglion cell axons and blood vessels in the region of the optic disc (**optic atrophy, Aa**). The disk becomes pale as a result.

- Anastomoses sometimes develop between the vessels on the disk and those of the peripapillary choroid due to chronic optic nerve compression (e. g., with slowly progressing optic nerve tumors) (**opticociliary shunt vessels, Aa**).

- Compression of the globe from behind can produce folding of the choroid (**choroid folds, Ab**). These choroid folds are usually arranged in parallel and are visible on funduscopy, but are seen even better on angiography. They tend to reduce visual function only slightly.

- More rarely, orbital tumors indent the globe (**globe indentation**), so that the appearance is that of an intraocular tumor.

- **Alterations of the lids,** such as retraction of the upper lid, are typical of endocrine orbitopathy but also occur in all forms of advanced exophthalmos. Swelling of the lacrimal gland often gives the upper lid lateral ptosis like an S-shape (**Ac**).

- Orbital diseases are often associated with **alterations of the conjunctiva**. Inflammatory conditions of the orbit usually and tumor processes occasionally cause redness (injection) and swelling (chemosis) of the conjunctiva. Carotid-cavernous sinus fistulas are characterized by dilatation of conjunctival and episcleral vessels because of the raised orbital venous pressure.

- There can be an **increase in intraocular pressure** as the aqueous humor is drained into the orbital veins. Compression of these veins sometimes leads to congestion of the aqueous humor and so to an increase in ocular pressure. An abnormality of venous orbital outflow with ocular hypertension is typical of carotid-cavernous sinus fistulas. In endocrine orbitopathy, there can be an increase in pressure depending on the direction of gaze ("pseudo-glaucoma").

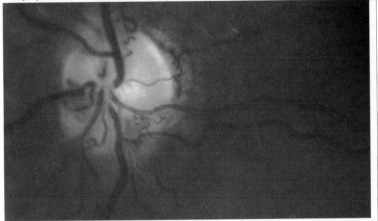

a Temporal pallor of the optic nerve (optic atrophy) and shunt vessels in optic glioma

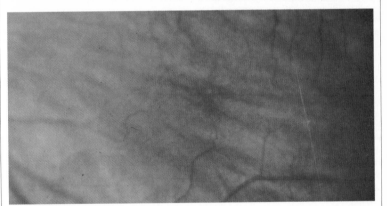

b Choroid folds running largely parallel in orbital metastasis

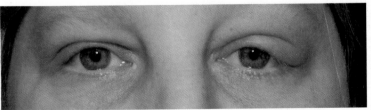

c Inflammation of the lacrimal gland (dacryoadenitis) on the left with typical S-shape

A. Investigations of Orbital Processes

The diagnosis begins with the history and clinical examination. Depending on these findings, imaging procedures are employed.

History. Obtaining an accurate history often provides valuable diagnostic hints. An inquiry is made about the development (acute or slow), the duration and nature of the symptoms, pain (inflammation is usually painful, tumors are usually not painful), and any previous injury.

Clinical examination. The eye is examined in bright light and with the slit lamp, and the examination also includes measurement of exophthalmos with the Hertel exophthalmometer. Anteriorly located processes should be palpated where possible to determine their consistency. Crackling subcutaneous emphysema on palpation is suggestive of a fracture of the ethmoid cells.

Examination of function. Simple tests used in the functional investigation of diseases of the orbit include measurement of visual acuity, the position and mobility of the eyes, and examination of pupillary reaction (swinging flashlight test). Examination of the visual field (perimetry) is usually also necessary. A reduction or loss of sensation in the area of distribution of the infraorbital nerve with a corresponding history indicates a fracture of the orbital floor. Occasionally, more complex diagnostic procedures are required such as measurement of the visual evoked potentials (VEP).

Imaging procedures (Aa–f). Processes located in the anterior orbit are readily accessible to ultrasound. This can be used to measure the thickness of the extrinsic ocular muscles, optic nerve sheath, and sclera and the extent and consistency of tumors, and to detect foreign bodies. Conditions at the apex of the orbit can also be imaged with computed tomography (CT) and magnetic resonance imaging (MRI). As a rule, orbital soft-tissue processes can be imaged better with MRI, and primary or secondary changes in the orbital bone better with CT. The circulatory relationships in the orbit (e.g., in carotid-cavernous sinus fistulas) can be examined using color duplex Doppler ultrasound. Angiography can be indicated in certain cases.

Biopsy. If an orbital process cannot be classified on the basis of the clinical and imaging investigations, a biopsy should be taken by fine-needle or excisional biopsy, at least when there is a progressive condition suggestive of malignancy. If a mixed tumor of the lacrimal gland (pleomorphic adenoma) is suspected, the entire lacrimal gland should be removed as an incisional biopsy in this situation is associated with an increased risk of recurrence.

B. Malformations

Malformations of the orbit are relatively rare apart from dermoid cysts. Defects of the sphenoid bone are sometimes found in neurofibromatosis. If the development of the bony orbit is abnormal, the meninges or brain can prolapse into the orbit (meningocele or encephalomeningocele). In Crouzon disease (craniofacial dysostosis) there is a narrow, shallow orbit so that the eyes protrude. Papilledema and optic atrophy can occur because of optic nerve compression. Orbital changes also form part of the mandibulofacial dysplasias such as Goldenhar, Rubinstein-Taybi or Hallermann-Streiff syndromes.

A. Investigations of Orbital Processes

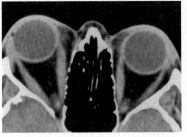

a CT in endocrine orbitopathy; marked thickening of the horizontal ocular muscles bilaterally

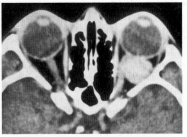

b CT of a retrobulbar cavernous hemangioma on the left

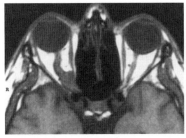

c MRI of an optic sheath meningioma in the region of the orbital apex on the right

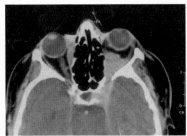

d CT of a non-Hodgkin lymphoma (NHL) in the region of the orbital apex on the left

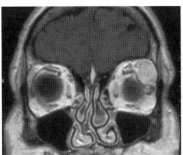

e MRI of a lacrimal gland tumor on the left

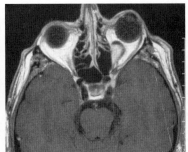

f MRI of a markedly dilated orbital vein (orbital varix) on the left, exophthalmos

A. Vascular Anomalies

Carotid-cavernous sinus fistulas are characterized by a pathological shunt between the arterial and venous system. This usually occurs spontaneously in older persons, and in younger persons it is mainly due to cranial trauma. The great increase in orbital venous pressure leads to congestion of venous blood (sometimes with reversed flow) and of aqueous humor. The typical findings therefore are dilated vessels and an increase in ocular pressure. The patient often notices a sound that is synchronous with the pulse, which can also be heard by the physician when the stethoscope is placed on the temple. Exophthalmos synchronous with the pulse is also typical. The treatment is determined by the extent of the disease. Smaller fistulas often close spontaneously. Fistulas that threaten vision or even life are closed by the neuroradiologist through a catheter.

Orbital varices (see p. 43, **Af**) usually occur without an identifiable cause. The patients notice exophthalmos, which increases during the Valsalva maneuver or when the head is lowered. Treatment is not usually necessary.

B. Inflammatory Conditions

Orbital cellulitis (**Ba** and **b**). This is a bacterial infection, which usually spreads from the paranasal sinuses into the orbit, or occurring more rarely after an open injury or as a result of a furuncle on the face. The commonest bacteria are staphylococci, streptococci, and *Haemophilus* species. The clinical picture is characterized by severe general malaise, exophthalmos, a motility deficit, and usually considerable lid and conjunctival swelling. Along with persistent loss of function due to damage to the optic nerve, there is sometimes a risk of cavernous sinus thrombosis leading to death. The treatment consists of prompt broad-spectrum antibiotics and often débridement of the paranasal sinuses. Subperiosteal abscesses of the orbit usually have to be drained.

Fungal infections of the orbit (*Aspergillus, Mucor/Mucorales*) have a less-fulminant course than bacterial infections but they are rather more difficult to treat. People with a compromised immune system are affected almost exclusively.

Orbital pseudotumor (**Bc**). This acute inflammation of orbital structures, probably of immunological origin, often affects the muscles (**myositis**). The very painful, usually unilateral disease responds very quickly and well to long-term corticosteroids. Recurrences and a variable course are not unusual.

Vasculitis such as Wegener disease or polyarteritis nodosa can be associated with orbital involvement.

Endocrine orbitopathy (**Bd**; see p. 43, **Aa**). This orbital inflammation is usually associated with autoimmune hyperthyroidism. The classical symptom triad of exophthalmos, goiter, and tachycardia (Merseburger triad) was described by Karl von Basedow/Robert Graves, so that the disease is also known as Basedow/Graves disease. It is very much more common in women than in men and commences acutely or subacutely. If it is untreated, there is spontaneous (partial) remission or transition to a scar stage. The symptoms are exophthalmos, which is usually bilateral, retraction, especially of the upper lids, and edema of the lids and conjunctiva. The commonest lid signs bear the name of their describers, von Graefe (lid lag when looking downward), Dalrymple (visible sclera at the upper border of the cornea), and Stellwag (reduction in the rate of blinking). There is often a motility deficit and strabismus, and exposure keratitis and optic nerve compression occur only in severe cases of the disease. The pressure of the thickened muscles on the globe on looking upward often causes a rise in ocular pressure ("pseudo-glaucoma"). In treatment, thyroid function must first be normalized. The inflammation is treated with corticosteroids. Immunosuppression is sometimes necessary. If loss of function due to optic nerve compression threatens, resection of orbital fat or opening of the paranasal sinuses must be performed to decompress the optic nerve. Cosmetic correction is performed in the noninflamed state.

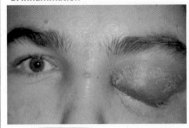

a Orbital cellulitis, massive swelling, and erythema of the upper lid

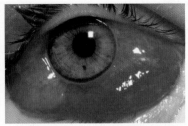

b Orbital cellulitis, massive swelling of the conjunctiva with hemorrhage beneath; exophthalmos, limited mobility of the globe

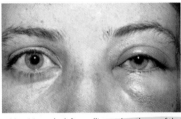

c Myositis on the left; swelling and erythema of the upper and lower lids

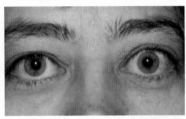

d Endocrine orbitopathy with exophthalmos particularly marked on the left; retraction of the upper lid with visible sclera at the upper border of the cornea (Dalrymple's sign)

A. Tumors

The spectrum of orbital tumors is markedly different in children from that in adults, and benign and malignant tumors occur at every age (**A, Table 1**). The commonest malignant orbital tumor in childhood is the **rhabdomyosarcoma** (**Aa**), which is characterized by rapid growth and an often inflammatory appearance. A biopsy confirms the diagnosis. The chances of cure are very good after adequate therapy, which consists of chemotherapy and radiotherapy.

Benign **dermoid cysts**, which arise from skin dermis displaced deeply, are located preferentially at the upper temporal entrance of the orbit. Not infrequently there are strands of tissue between the cyst and bony structures. Dermoid cysts are bordered by stratified keratinized squamous epithelium and filled with masses of keratin, sometimes containing hair. There are skin appendages (hairs and sebaceous glands) and not rarely inflammatory infiltrates in the region of the cyst wall. Complete surgical excision is usually done before the child starts school. **Hemangiomas** (**Ab**) and **lymphangiomas** of the orbit in children are usually operated only when visual function is endangered due to amblyopia (e.g., due to tumor-induced ptosis) or optic nerve compression. **Optic nerve glioma**, occasionally occurring in neurofibromatosis (see p. 39, **Aa**, and p. 41, **Aa**), and **optic sheath meningioma** (see p. 43, **Ac**) very often cause considerable losses of function despite being biologically benign. Surgical excision usually leads to deterioration in function on the affected side but can be indicated to prevent growth of the tumor into the chiasm and the opposite side. Tumors of the optic nerve can be irradiated successfully.

In adults, the commonest primary malignant tumors are **non-Hodgkin lymphoma** (**NHL**, see p. 43, **Ad**), adenoid cystic lacrimal gland carcinoma, which is often associated with severe pain because of nerve infiltration, and malignant fibrous histiocytoma.

However, **metastases** from breast, bronchial, prostate, and gastrointestinal carcinomas and from cutaneous melanomas are commoner than primary malignancies (**Ac** and p. 41, **Ab**); orbital invasion from carcinomas of the paranasal sinuses, the lacrimal sac, and especially malignant tumors of the lids and conjunctiva (basal cell carcinoma, squamous cell carcinoma, conjunctival melanoma) also occur. Both in children (retinoblastoma) and in adults (malignant choroid melanoma), primary intraocular tumors can perforate the sclera and mimic an orbital tumor through intraorbital growth. Occasionally (sphenoid) meningiomas grow into the orbit from inside the skull. Outpouchings of the paranasal sinus mucosa (mucocele) into the orbit can give the impression of an orbital tumor.

The treatment of malignant orbital tumors in adults, depending on the type and extent of the neoplasm, consists of radiation, surgical excision, or exenteration of the orbit, where the entire orbital contents including the globe and periosteum are removed (**Ad**). Benign tumors of the orbit can be observed if function is normal and progression does not occur.

A. Tumors

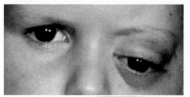

a Rhabdomyosarcoma of the left orbit with considerable inferior displacement of the eye; slightly inflammatory appearance of the upper and lower lid

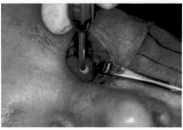

b Cryoextraction of an orbital hemangioma located nasally above the globe

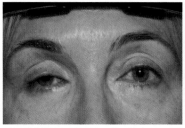

c Enophthalmos on the right with orbital metastasis from breast cancer

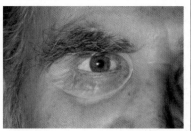

d Treatment of a facial defect by an epithesis following exenteration of the orbit

Table 1 Orbital tumors in childhood and adulthood

	Childhood	Adulthood
Benign	Dermoid cyst, hemangioma (capillary), lymphangioma, optic glioma, juvenile xanthogranuloma (JXG), eosinophilic granuloma (rare), Langerhans cell histiocytosis, orbital teratoma (very rare), others	Pseudotumor of the orbit, hemangioma (cavernous), fibrous histiocytoma, fibroma, neurinoma, neurofibroma, dermoid cyst, pleomorphic adenoma of the lacrimal gland, optic sheath meningioma, optic glioma, fibrous dysplasia, osteoma, hemangiopericytoma, intracranial meningioma with orbital invasion, others
Malignant, primary	Rhabdomyosarcoma, neuroblastoma	Non-Hodgkin lymphoma (NHL), adenoid cystic carcinoma of the lacrimal gland, malignant fibrous histiocytoma, rhabdomyosarcoma (very rare), malignant melanoma (very rare)
Malignant, secondary	Retinoblastoma with orbital invasion, leukemic infiltrates, metastases (rather rare)	Tumors of the lids and conjunctiva with orbital invasion (basal cell carcinoma, melanoma, squamous cell carcinoma), malignant melanoma of the choroid with orbital invasion, malignancies of the paranasal sinuses with orbital invasion, plasmacytoma (rare), leukemic infiltrates (rare), lacrimal sac carcinoma with orbital invasion (very rare)

A. Injuries

Blunt force to the eye, e.g., due to sports balls or a blow from a fist, lead to brief but considerable compression of the orbital soft tissues. As a result of the increase in intraorbital pressure, fracture of the thin orbital bone in the region of the orbital lamina of the ethmoid and especially of the orbital floor often occurs (**"blow-out fracture," Aa** and **b**). Orbital floor fractures are often associated with a loss of sensation in the area of distribution of the infraorbital nerve. If tissue is incarcerated in the wound gap, enophthalmos and a motility deficit are often found. Subcutaneous emphysema, which is usually characterized by the typical sensation on palpation in the region of the lids, is typical of fractures in the region of the ethmoid cells. Fractures of the orbit without significant bone dehiscence, enophthalmos, and motility deficit do not always have to be operated. However, systemic antibiotics and a prohibition on sneezing are recommended in order to prevent penetration of bacteria from the paranasal sinuses into the orbit. Fractures of the orbital floor associated with greater tissue prolapse are treated surgically, usually by insertion of a plate.

Traumatic hematomas of the orbit have to be decompressed surgically if significant compression of the optic nerve is present (examination of pupil reactions). In these cases there is usually massively increased lid tension. Midface fractures occur not infrequently in conjunction with head injuries. If the fracture line passes through the optic canal as in LeFort II and LeFort III fractures, there is a danger of injury to the optic nerve by bone fragments or overstretching (**traumatic optic neuropathy**). However, stretching of the optic nerve can also occur in the region of the optic canal in the absence of a fracture. The decision on treatment is difficult as neither high-dose corticosteroids nor surgical decompression of the optic nerve canal has yielded convincing results.

The extent of penetrating injuries of the orbit (**Ac**) is often underestimated. There can often be a major optic nerve injury even when the external wound is small. Penetration of a foreign body into the orbit and penetration of the globe must always also be considered. Operative wound management may be required depending on the situation. Organic **foreign bodies** in particular should be removed as they otherwise usually cause a severe inflammatory reaction. Foreign bodies made of certain metals (most forms of steel, silver, gold, aluminum), glass, or porcelain can sometimes be left in the orbit as they normally do not cause any significant tissue reaction.

B. Systematic Classification

The flow chart in **B** opposite shows the systematic classification of all orbital diseases.

A. Injuries

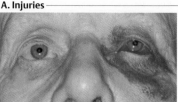

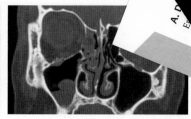

a Fracture of the floor of the left orbit with lid hematoma and subconjunctival hemorrhage

b CT of a fracture of the right orbital floor and medial orbital wall; opacity of the maxillary sinus and ethmoid cells due to hemorrhage

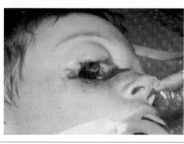

c Penetrating injury of the orbit due to a tree branch which had penetrated as far as the region of the cavernous sinus and had divided the optic nerve

B. Systematic Classification

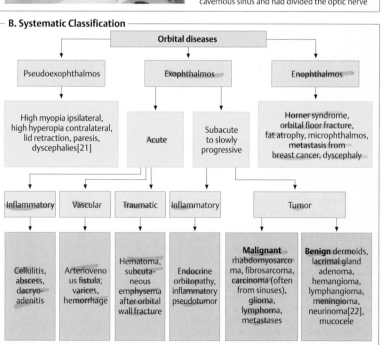

```
                        Orbital diseases
       ┌────────────────────┼────────────────────┐
Pseudoexophthalmos      Exophthalmos          Enophthalmos
```

Pseudoexophthalmos	Exophthalmos		Enophthalmos
High myopia ipsilateral, high hyperopia contralateral, lid retraction, paresis, dyscephalies[21]	Acute	Subacute to slowly progressive	Horner syndrome, orbital floor fracture, fat atrophy, microphthalmos, metastasis from breast cancer, dyscephaly

Inflammatory	Vascular	Traumatic	Inflammatory	Tumor	
Cellulitis, abscess, dacryoadenitis	Arteriovenous fistula, varices, hemorrhage	Hematoma, subcutaneous emphysema after orbital wall fracture	Endocrine orbitopathy, inflammatory pseudotumor	**Malignant** rhabdomyosarcoma, fibrosarcoma, carcinoma (often from sinuses), glioma, lymphoma, metastases	**Benign** dermoids, lacrimal gland adenoma, hemangioma, lymphangioma, meningioma, neurinoma[22], mucocele

Definition

Errors of eye alignment are called strabismus (squint, heterotropia). Along with eye alignment, visual acuity, refraction, fixation, motility, and stereoscopic vision play a part in diagnosis.

B. Tests of Visual Acuity

In children, tests of visual acuity are possible from the second year of life at the earliest. Prior to that, the preferential use of one eye and reduced visual acuity of the other can be examined by covering one eye. On occlusion of the better-seeing eye (**occlusion test**), a defensive reaction occurs. Other methods of assessing visual acuity in infants include holding up a 10 cm/m vertical prism, producing **optokinetic nystagmus** (OKN) and the **preferential looking test** with Teller striated pattern charts. Löhlein child pictures or the **LH test** (Lea Hyvärinen test) can be used in children over 2 years. Near acuity is tested with Landolt rings at a test distance of 30 cm.

Decreased visual acuity may be evidence of **amblyopia** if further investigation excludes an organic cause for the reduction in acuity. Amblyopia is regarded as a diagnosis of exclusion. It is defined as visual weakness in an otherwise normal eye (**B**).

C. Examination of Eye Alignment

An orientating examination of eye alignment can be performed using the corneal light reflection (**Hirschberg test, Ca**). Exact assessment is made possible by the unilateral cover test and alternating covering and uncovering (with and without prisms) in which the patient fixes on a visual object at a defined distance. In the unilateral cover test, the examiner covers the apparently fixating eye and observes the movement of the other eye (**Cb**). If an adjustment movement occurs, **manifest strabismus** (heterotropia) is present. No adjustment movement is observed when there is either no squint (**orthotropia**) or if the squinting eye was covered. Adjustment movements during the **alternating cover test** indicate **latent strabismus** (heterophoria). If the eye that was covered last makes a slow fusional movement on uncovering, that is, during binocular vision, this suggests good function. When the prism is held up with a strength corresponding to the objective squint angle, no further adjustment movement occurs. The tip of the prism points in the direction of the squint. Poor cooperation (lack of fixation) and eccentric fixation (see below) limit assessment of the unilateral cover test.

D. Examination of Fixation

The best possible visual acuity is obtained only with foveal (= central) fixation. If, on the other hand, a different part of the retina is used for fixation (eccentric fixation), the visual acuity falls depending on the distance from the fovea (**D**). Fixation is a monocular process, so central fixation can exist even in the presence of a squint. During binocular vision central fixation of one eye is given up and anomalous retinal correspondence (ARC) results. Central fixation and ARC are thus not mutually exclusive. Examination of fixation is always monocular. For instance, the position of the corneal reflection image can be assessed. It is better to examine fixation with a visuscope. This is an ophthalmoscope with a 1° sized test mark that is reproduced on the patient's macula. The patient is asked to fixate on this mark and the examiner can then assess the position of the mark on the retina. As well as the location of the fixation point, the type of fixation, e.g., smooth, unsteady, or nystagmic, is assessed.

B. Test of Visual Acuity

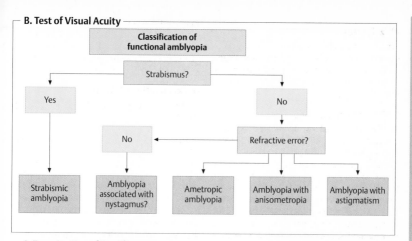

Classification of functional amblyopia

Strabismus?

Yes → Strabismic amblyopia

No → Refractive error?

No → Amblyopia associated with nystagmus?

Ametropic amblyopia

Amblyopia with anisometropia

Amblyopia with astigmatism

C. Examination of Eye Alignment

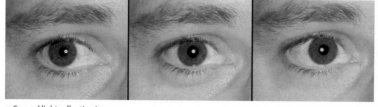

a Corneal light reflection images

D. Examination of Fixation

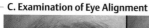

Foveal

Parafoveal

Paramacular

Parapapillary

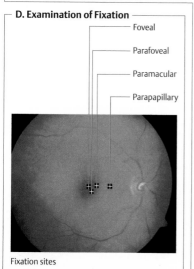

Fixation sites

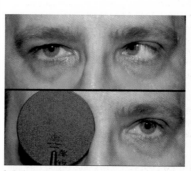

b Unilateral cover test

A. Examination of Retinal Correspondence

Examination for normal (NRC) or anomalous retinal correspondence (ARC) is important in the investigation of binocular vision (**Aa**). The **Bagolini striated glass test** (light trail test) is most often employed. When one is looking at a fixation light through fine parallel grooves scratched or etched onto glass, a streak of light perpendicular to the grooves on the glass is perceived because of the light scattering. When the grooves on both lenses are arranged by moving them by 90° (e. g. at an angle of 135° on the right and 45° on the left) the normal patient perceives a light cross with the fixation light at the site where they cross. Fusion is impaired only slightly in this test as the surroundings continue to be seen through the lenses. The patient is asked to describe how they see the light streaks and the light source (**Ab**). The Bagolini light streak test investigates binocular vision and retinal correspondence can be examined when cooperation is good. Another test of correspondence is the **Hering afterimage**, which can be used in central fixation. With a flashing device, different images (e. g. a horizontal and a vertical bar) are flashed into each eye onto the fixation site. The patient then describes the relationship of the two afterimages to each other, which in each case represents the direction of the fovea of each eye. If the position of the afterimages is reported at the same site (e. g. a cross in the middle), then both foveas have the same spatial perception independent of the eye alignment. There is thus normal retinal correspondence (NRC). If the afterimages are in different sites, there is **anomalous** retinal correspondence (ARC).

B. Examination of Binocular Vision

Simultaneous vision, fusion, and stereoscopic vision are distinguished in binocular vision. If horizontally disparate images separated by color or polarization are offered to the two eyes, these images can be fused into one image with depth perception if stereoscopic vision is present. **Stereopsis** can be quantified by grading the horizontal disparity. Common tests of stereoscopic vision tests used as sample images are the **Lang stereo test**, the **Titmus test** and the **TNO test**. The Lang test does not require glasses and can therefore be used as a screening test even in small children to exclude a squint.

C. Measurement of the squint angle

The subjective squint angle can be measured with the **dark red glass test** with appropriate cooperation. When a dark red glass is held in front of one eye, **fusion** (merging of two visual impressions into one image) is abolished. Different images are thus perceived with the two eyes, and the examiner enquires about their positions relative to each other. Reliable statements are obtained only when there is normal retinal correspondence (NRC) and central fixation. The patient fixates on a light source that is located in the middle of a tangential table or on the **Harms tangent wall**. When one eye is covered with the dark red glass, the patient now perceives only a red point of light with the covered eye. Through the brain, the patient localizes the red light point to the corresponding retinal site of the other eye, i. e. to its fovea. With normal eye alignment, the red light point and the yellow fixation light can now be perceived alternately (**confusion**). In the case of heterotropia or heterophoria, the red light point is not localized in the center of the tangent table. The patient can establish the subjective squint angle by stating the site where they perceive the red light point. If instead of a fixation light a light strip is used, the axis of which can be adjusted, the deviation of the eyes relative to each other (**cyclotropia**) can be measured.

A. Examination of Retinal Correspondence

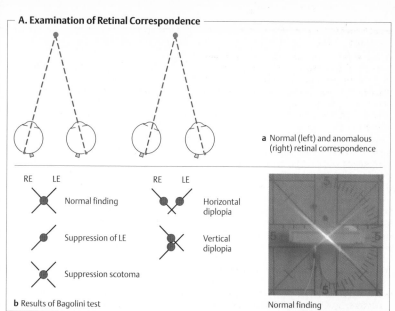

a Normal (left) and anomalous (right) retinal correspondence

RE   LE

✱ Normal finding

✱ Suppression of LE

✱ Suppression scotoma

RE   LE

✱ Horizontal diplopia

✱ Vertical diplopia

b Results of Bagolini test

Normal finding

C. Measurement of Squint Angle

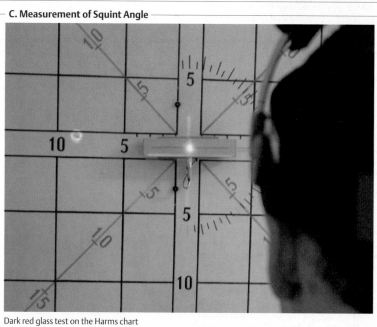

Dark red glass test on the Harms chart

A. Examination of Eye Movement

Strabismus is often associated with a disorder of eye motility. As an orientating test, the position of the eyes relative to each other is examined during slow following movements (**examination of eye motility according to pursuit movements**) in the nine diagnostically important directions of gaze (**Aa**). Deviation in the final positions of each of these nine gaze directions and a change in the squint angle in different positions of gaze (**incomitant strabismus**) can be examined using the position of the corneal reflection images and the cover test (**Ab**). When the squint angle is the same in the different directions of gaze, we speak of **concomitant strabismus**. The squint angle can be quantified with the unilateral and alternating prism cover test and the dark red glass test (see above).

Other examination methods that are used to elucidate **supranuclear disorders of eye movement** are examination of saccades, examination of pursuit movement and optokinetic nystagmus, and examination of the vestibulo-ocular reflex (VOR). **Saccades** are rapid eye movements by which the fovea is directed quickly toward certain visual objects. The innervation pattern required for them is generated in the **reticular formation** of the brainstem. Two visual targets are offered to the patient (e. g., the ends of a rod ca. 15 cm long) at a distance of about 50 cm. The patient is then told to fix the ends of the rod alternately as quickly as possible on command. Saccades can be slowed or inaccurate, i. e., too short (hypometric) or too long (hypermetric). Pathological changes are found with paralysis of the ocular muscles or in diseases that involve the supranuclear control of eye movement. **Slow pursuit movements** of the eyes serve to produce a continuous foveal image of moving visual objects so that they are always identified sharply. **Optokinetic nystagmus** is triggered when a striped pattern is moved before the patient's eyes. Looking at the landscape from the window of a moving train also produces optokinetic nystagmus. The slow phase of the nystagmus is used for keeping the eyes on the target and thus ensuring a sharp image, while the fast phase brings the eyes back to the starting position.

B. Classification

The **distinguishing characteristics** of the different errors of eye alignment are described according to the type of strabismus (convergent squint, divergent squint, vertical squint), the cause (paralytic, nonparalytic, secondary, consecutive), the degree (heterophoria, heterotropia), the location (unilateral, alternating), the temporal occurrence (constant, intermittent), and the size of the squint angle in different gaze positions (concomitant, incomitant). The most common distinction is between **paralytic** and **nonparalytic** squint. Further findings such as amblyopia, anomalous head posture, and nystagmus are also employed for description. **Manifest squint** is the term used when a squint is present constantly. **Latent squint** occurs only under certain examination conditions and is not present during normal conditions of binocular vision. **Intermittent squint** is present when a squint occurs only occasionally.

In **nonparalytic squint** the function of the ocular muscles is not impaired, so that the squint angle is about the same in all directions (**concomitant strabismus**). The cause is probably absent or delayed development of the nerve cells in the brain that control binocular vision. A permanent disorder of binocular vision results. In order to suppress double image perception, adaptation mechanisms such as **suppression** of one image and development of **anomalous retinal correspondence** are used by the child's brain.

A. Examination of Eye Movement

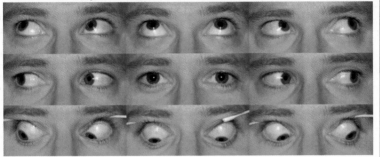

a The nine diagnostic gaze directions

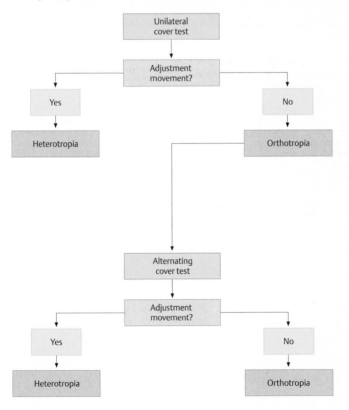

b Examination of eye alignment with the unilateral and alternating cover tests

A. Early infantile Convergent Strabismus (Esotropia)

Convergent strabismus occurs within the first six months of life and is the most common form of squint. The squint angle is often nearly equal on distant and near vision and is independent of the direction of gaze. There is convergence excess when the squint angle is much greater on near vision than when looking into the distance. If the near angle can be compensated by plus glasses to provide further near addition, this is called accommodative convergence excess (**Aa, b**) Hyperopia is usually present and amblyopia is also present in the case of unilateral squint. In addition, **latent nystagmus** develops and a vertical squint (**supraduction** and/or **dissociated vertical squint**) is observed. The treatment is prescription of glasses when there is farsightedness and a high degree of astigmatism. Otherwise, **occlusion** of the fixating eye is indicated with unilateral squint. After good visual acuity is achieved, surgery can be performed on the ocular muscles to improve eye alignment. Even when treatment commences early, normal binocular vision (high-quality stereopsis) cannot be achieved. The aim of treatment is good bilateral visual acuity and inconspicuous eye alignment.

B. Normosensorial Essential Late Strabismus

Normosensorial late strabismus is the term for a convergent squint that typically occurs only between the ages of 2 and 4 years. The squint angle is smaller than in infantile strabismus. The children may report double vision or may close one eye. The squint can be intermittent initially. There is normal retinal correspondence. If a refraction error is present, this is usually hyperopia, and glasses are prescribed first therapeutically. If the convergent squint persists despite the glasses, an ocular muscle operation should be performed as soon as possible in order to prevent amblyopia and a loss of binocular vision (stereopsis). The prognosis in normosensorial strabismus is good when surgery is performed in time as it can be assumed that there was normal binocular cooperation before the onset of the squint.

C. Microstrabismus

Microstrabismus is the term for a convergent squint with a squint angle below 5°. The squint angle is not noticeable cosmetically, making it difficult to discover the eye misalignment and favoring the development of amblyopia. Often the squint is only discovered at the school entry examination due to an absence of stereopsis. There is anomalous retinal correspondence and there is also often eccentric fixation of the deviating eye. Thus, amblyopia is also observed regularly. The treatment consists of occlusion of the eye with better vision in order to treat the amblyopia. Normal binocular vision cannot be achieved even with successful treatment of the amblyopia. If the microstrabismus is discovered after the age of 6 or 7 years, normal visual acuity usually cannot be achieved in the deviating eye despite intensive occlusion.

D. Intermittent Divergent Strabismus (Exotropia)

Intermittent divergent squint (**D**) is less common than convergent squint. With intermittent divergent squint the deviation of the eye is usually not noticed by the patient. The intermittent divergent squint becomes more frequent when the patient is fatigued and in poor general condition. The squint usually starts at the age of 2 or 3 years, and amblyopia is rare. A squint operation can be performed if the squint is frequent and noticeable, but complete elimination of the divergent squint is seldom achieved and recurrences of a newly noticeable divergent squint can occur.

E. Consecutive Divergent Strabismus

A previously existing convergent squint changes into a divergent squint spontaneously or after an operation. There is no binocular vision. If the squint is noticeable, eye alignment can be improved with ocular muscle surgery.

A. Early Infantile Convergent Strabismus (Esotropia)

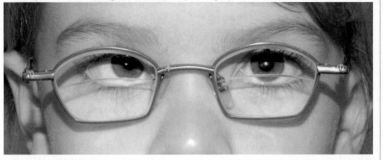

a Convergent strabismus with convergence excess (fixation through distance segments)

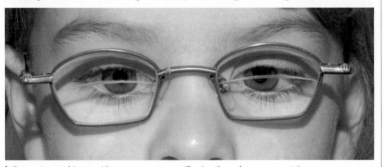

b Convergent strabismus with convergence excess (fixation through near segments)

D. Intermittent Divergent Strabismus (Exotropia)

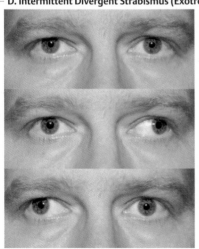

A. Secondary Divergent Strabismus

The divergent squint occurs after prolonged visual impairment of an eye. The squint angle increases gradually over years. Eye alignment can be improved by ocular muscle surgery.

B. Associated Forms of Strabismus

These forms of squint can occur in conjunction with a horizontal error of eye alignment, usually with early childhood convergent squint. In **A or V pattern strabismus** (**Ba**) the lines traced by the two eyes when looking up and down form an A or a V, i. e. the horizontal squint angle changes on looking up or down. A disorder in the equilibrium between the tensile forces of the oblique ocular muscles (e. g., underfunctioning of the inferior oblique in A incomitancy) causes this incomitancy. In **dissociated vertical divergence** (**Bb, c**) the eye that is not fixating drifts upward. If the fixation changes, then the vertical squint changes to the other eye. **Strabismus sursoadductorius** (**Bd**) is the term used when the adducting eye is higher on looking to the side. This form of squint is often associated with V incomitancy and there is usually overfunctioning of the inferior oblique muscle. Unilateral strabismus sursoadductorius can also be a sign of fourth nerve palsy.

C. Latent Heterophoria

When fusion is interrupted, e. g., during the alternating cover test, an adjustment movement of the uncovered eye can be observed in about 80% of the population. Horizontal, or more rarely vertical, deviation occurs, which is described as heterophoria, e. g., esophoria with convergent strabismus. When there is binocular vision again, the phoria is compensated by fusion. Heterophoria becomes pathological only when **asthenopic symptoms** occur during fusion efforts or when the deviation can no longer be fused. Heterophoria can decompensate particularly when there is physical or mental stress and under the effect of medications or alcohol. Treatment first involves correction of any refractive errors. If the symptoms persist, the heterophoria can be improved by prescribing prisms. Squint angles greater than 6° are corrected by ocular muscle surgery.

D. Paralytic Strabismus

Paralytic squint is a disorder of ocular muscle function in the form of **palsy** or complete **paralysis**. The cause is located in the orbit, the cavernous sinus, the posterior cranial fossa, or the supratentorial region. If several cranial nerves are affected, there is usually a lesion in the cavernous sinus or in the superior orbital fissure. In paralytic squint, the squint angle and the distance between the double images depends on the direction of gaze (incomitancy) with the greatest angle on gaze in the direction of pull of the affected ocular muscle. The squint angle is smaller (**primary squint angle**) on fixation with the healthy eye than on fixation with the affected eye (**secondary squint angle**). Along with the eye misalignment and the motility disorder, an anomalous head posture is often adopted to minimize the double vision. The head is turned in the direction of the main function of the paralytic muscle. Paralytic squint is more common in adults than in children. The most important causes are circulatory disorders, head injury, compression due to a space-occupying lesion, and inflammation. The differential diagnosis includes congenital disorders of eye movement and muscle diseases. As palsies can resolve, **conservative therapy** is indicated initially. Troublesome double vision is eliminated by covering with **translucent tape** or by prisms. An operation is performed when the findings remain constant (usually after a year). The aim of the operation is the largest possible visual field with simple binocular vision and without anomalous head posture.

B. Associated Forms of Strabismus

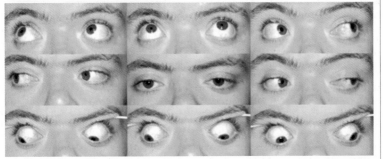

a A-pattern

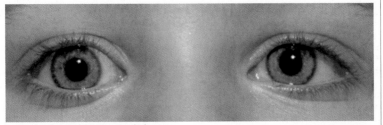

b Dissociated vertical divergence, right fixation

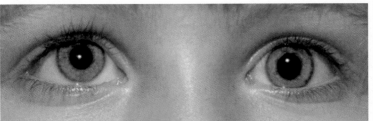

c Dissociated vertical divergence, left fixation

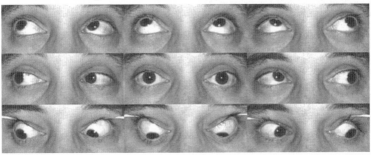

d Strabismus sursoadductorius

A. Sixth Nerve (Abducent Nerve) Palsy

Partial or complete paralysis of the lateral rectus muscle leads to an incomitant convergent squint (**Aa**). In adults the palsy often occurs with cerebral circulatory disorders in diabetes mellitus and arterial hypertension. Head injury with stretching of the sixth cranial nerve and a space-occupying lesion in the course of the nerve along with inflammatory conditions and indirect injury because of raised cerebrospinal fluid pressure are further causes. In children, sixth nerve palsy is caused more often by an intracerebral space-occupying lesion. Trauma, inflammation and rarely pseudoinfections after immunization are further causes. The clinical symptom is sudden-onset double vision with the images side by side. When the paresis is very slight, the complaint is often only of indistinct vision. The distance between the double images is greater at a distance than near, and is greatest on looking toward the affected side. Sometimes the head is turned toward the side of the affected eye. The abduction saccade is markedly slowed. Other neurological symptoms (ipsilateral facial palsy, ipsilateral loss of sensation in the area innervated by the trigeminal nerve, and/or contralateral hemiparesis) are signs of a lesion of the abducent nucleus region in the brainstem. In the differential diagnosis, especially in children, the **retraction syndrome** (Stilling-Türk-Duane, **Ab**) should be considered. This is a congenital disorder of ocular movement with a large variety of clinical variants. The cause is hypoplasia of the abducent nucleus and growth of oculomotor fibers into the lateral rectus muscle. Abduction is most commonly affected, but adduction can also be restricted. Because of the co-innervation of the lateral rectus and medial rectus muscles, eyeball retraction with narrowing of the lid fissure occurs on adduction. The disorder is usually unilateral and an anomalous head posture is adopted.

B. Fourth Nerve (Trochlear Nerve) Palsy

Corresponding to the main action of the superior oblique muscle (inward deviation, depression on adduction), vertical oblique double vision with image deviation occurs with unilateral fourth nerve paresis. The distance between the double images is particularly great on looking downward in adduction (e. g., when reading or climbing stairs). Compensatory head tilting occurs: the head is tilted to the side of the healthy eye, the face is turned to the affected side, and the chin is lowered. The affected eye is higher than the healthy one on adduction (supraduction), the hypertropia and the excyclotropia also become greater on lowering the gaze (**B**). The convergent deviation that also occurs becomes greater on looking down (V incomitancy), because the abducting action of the superior oblique muscle is missing. The **Bielschowsky phenomenon** is important diagnostically; when the head is tilted to the affected side, the higher position of the paralytic eye increases and it diminishes when the head is tilted to the healthy side.

With bilateral fourth nerve palsy, strabismus is usually not apparent, but the patient perceives tilted double images because of the excyclotropy. The outward deviation is greater on looking down than in unilateral paresis (usually >10°). The V incomitancy is also usually greater with bilateral palsy than with unilateral. In the differential diagnosis, fourth nerve palsy must be distinguished from **strabismus sursoadductorius**, a congenital disorder. Here, too, the affected eye is higher on adduction but there is no increase in the angle on looking down.

A. Sixth Nerve Palsy

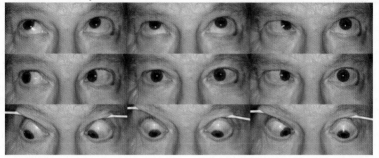

a Sixth nerve palsy on the left

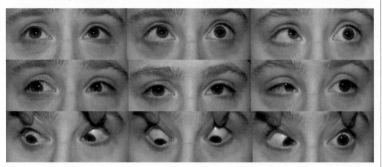

b Retraction syndrome on the left

B. Fourth Nerve Palsy

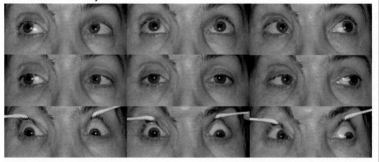

Fourth nerve palsy on the right

A. Third Nerve (Oculomotor Nerve) Palsy

Complete oculomotor nerve palsy (**Aa**) leads to ptosis, exotropia, and a major reduction in adduction, elevation, and depression. The pupil is dilated, the pupillary light reaction is reduced or abolished, and accommodation is paralyzed (**Ab**). If the pupil and accommodation are not affected, this is termed **external oculomotor nerve palsy**. It is often observed in circulatory disorders. Pupil dilatation occurs when the oculomotor nerve is compressed. Rarely, only a single oculomotor branch is affected. Particularly after traumatic oculomotor nerve palsy, aberrant regeneration can occur. For instance, nerve fibers from the medial rectus muscle can innervate the levator palpebrae muscle. The upper lid is then elevated on adduction. If there is pupillary involvement (mydriasis) or no resolution, a cranial CT or MRI should be performed. Depending on the extent of the affected ocular muscles, therapy with prisms should be prescribed, and after a healing period of 9–12 months ocular muscle surgery should be considered. Differential diagnoses include myasthenia, chronic progressive external ophthalmoplegia, endocrine orbitopathy, and orbital pseudotumor.

B. Complex Paralytic Strabismus

This includes diseases that are associated with paralytic squint. Various diseases at the apex of the orbit are grouped together as **orbital apex syndrome**, which lead to paralysis of all the nerves to the ocular muscles and the first division of the trigeminal nerve (V1). Important causes are arteriovenous fistulas, sinus venous thrombosis, inflammatory orbital diseases (cellulitis, mucormycosis and Tolosa-Hunt syndrome), and tumors. Exophthalmos is often observed with an orbital lesion. **Myasthenia gravis** is often first manifested in the eye; ptosis and alternating double vision are observed in the predominantly elderly patients. The complaints vary with the time of day, and the muscle weakness often becomes worse toward evening. Symptoms on speaking, swallowing, and breathing are signs of generalized involvement. The muscle function is improved briefly by intravenous injection of edrophonium chloride (e.g., Tensilon). **Chronic progressive external ophthalmoplegia** (**CPEO**) is a mitochondriopathy. There is slowly progressive weakness of all the ocular muscles with a variable degree of motility disorders and corresponding double vision, and subsequently there is also involvement of the limb muscles. Bilateral ptosis with greatly impaired levator function is often observed. In addition there is weakness of the muscles of facial expression, particularly the orbicularis oculi. A special form is the **Kearns-Sayre syndrome**. Along with the muscle weakness there are changes in the fundus like those of retinitis pigmentosa and also cardiac arrhythmias, hearing disorders, and mental retardation. Causal treatment of CPEO is not possible.

C. Mechanical Disorders

In orbital fractures, orbital structures can become trapped in the fracture and thus lead to a mechanical disorder of movement. This is found most often in fractures of the orbital floor. Elevation and depression are then impaired. There is often also a loss of sensation in the cheek and upper lip due to injury of the infraorbital nerve. In **Brown syndrome** the underlying cause is thickening of the superior oblique tendon and/or trochlea, which prevents the tendon from gliding through the trochlea (**C**). This interferes with the function of the inferior oblique muscle from a certain point of gaze excursion because of the fixed position of the superior oblique tendon in the trochlea. The causes are a congenital anomaly of the muscle tendon or trochlea or acquired changes after trauma, operation, and rheumatoid inflammation.

Third Nerve Palsy

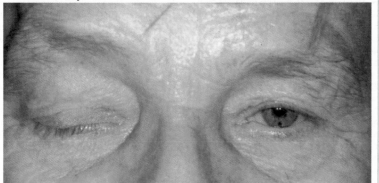

a Ptosis in complete third nerve palsy

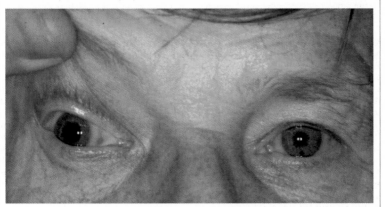

b Complete third nerve palsy with the lid held up, divergence, and mydriasis

C. Mechanical Disorders

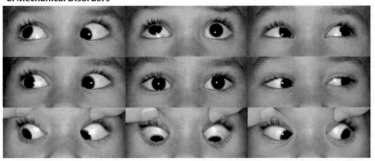

Brown syndrome on the left

A. Supranuclear Disorders of Eye Movement

These include disorders of coordinated eye movement caused by lesions of the neural structures proximal to the ocular muscle nuclei or of the tracts that link the ocular muscle nuclei with each other (**Aa**). **Gaze palsy** means disorders of movement of both eyes due to damage to the structures that control conjugate eye movements. Because of the proximity of the cranial nerve nuclei III, IV, and VI, gaze palsy is often combined with a paralytic squint. **Horizontal gaze palsy** can be caused by a lesion in the abducent nucleus or in the paramedian pontine reticular formation (**PPRF**). In a **lesion of the abducent nucleus**, all types of conjugate eye movements to the side of the lesion are disturbed. When there is **damage to the PPRF** only rapid ipsilateral directed eye movements are lost while pursuit movements and the vestibulo-ocular reflex are preserved. In acute lesions of the PPRF **tonic deviation of gaze** and spontaneous nystagmus to the opposite side are observed. A lesion in the **internal capsule** can cause a gaze palsy that usually disappears after two weeks. Gaze to the side opposite to the lesion is paralyzed and there is tonic deviation of gaze to the side of the lesion. Vertical gaze palsy can be grouped under the **Parinaud syndrome**. Isolated paralysis of upward gaze is often caused by a **pineal tumor**, which leads to interruption of the fibers that cross in the posterior commissure in the midbrain. The very rarely occurring isolated paralysis of downward gaze arises from a bilateral lesion of the **RIMLF** (rostral interstitial nucleus of the medial longitudinal fasciculus) through occlusion of the posterior thalamo-subthalamic artery. In the Parinaud syndrome, convergent nystagmus often occurs on looking upward. In addition, an **Argyll-Robertson pupil** is described in Parinaud syndrome. The light reaction is absent while the accommodation reaction is preserved.

Congenital **oculomotor apraxia** is called **Cogan syndrome**, in which the patient cannot voluntarily initiate horizontal saccades.

Internuclear ophthalmoplegia (INO) is the term for prenuclear paralysis of the medial rectus muscle. The affected eye cannot be adducted when the gaze direction is changed but can be by near accommodation convergence. The adduction saccade is markedly slowed in INO. There is often **directional nystagmus** to the side opposite the lesion. The cause of INO is a lesion of the excitatory internuclear neurons, which originate from the abducent nucleus, cross to the other side and ascend in the medial longitudinal fasciculus (MLF) to reach the subnucleus of the medial rectus muscle. Since there are also fibers in the MLF that are responsible for vertical eye movements, a vertical squint (skew deviation) can occasionally occur with INO. Moreover, the adjacent ipsilateral PPRF or the abducent nucleus can also be damaged along with the MLF. This produces the **one and a half syndrome**: horizontal motility in the ipsilateral eye is completely abolished (no adduction and abduction), but only adduction is paralyzed in the contralateral eye. A frequent cause of INO is multiple sclerosis. Differential diagnosis: myasthenia.

Damage to the graviceptive tracts (from the otolith apparatus to the ocular muscles and to the neck muscles and cerebral cortex) leads to the **ocular tilt reaction**. The following four abnormalities are observed: tilting of the subjective visual verticals; rotation of both eyes around the line of gaze (cycloduction); vertical strabismus; and head tilted to one shoulder (skew deviation). All four components show tilting in the same direction (**Ab–d**) Tilting to the same side is seen with a lesion in the region of the lower brainstem (medulla oblongata, lower pons) and to the opposite side with damage to the upper brainstem.

A. Supranuclear Disorders of Eye Movement

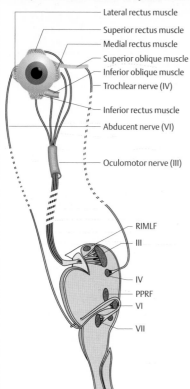

- Lateral rectus muscle
- Superior rectus muscle
- Medial rectus muscle
- Superior oblique muscle
- Inferior oblique muscle
- Trochlear nerve (IV)
- Inferior rectus muscle
- Abducent nerve (VI)
- Oculomotor nerve (III)
- RIMLF
- III
- IV
- PPRF
- VI
- VII

a Innervation of the extraocular eye muscles

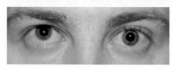

b Ocular tilt

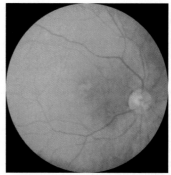

c Fundus of right eye: incyclorotation

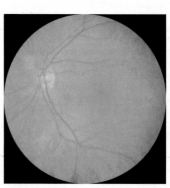

d Fundus of left eye: excyclorotation

A. Malformations

Microphthalmos (= small eye) and cryptophthalmos (= usually microphthalmic eye concealed by the absence of a palpebral fissure) are associated with an often massively reduced conjunctival sac, which makes it considerably difficult to fit an artificial eye. The **limbal dermoid** and the **lipodermoid** (**A**) that occurs in a superior temporal location are congenital tumors (choristomas) of the conjunctiva. Both can be associated with Goldenhar syndrome. The lipodermoid should be approached surgically with great care, if at all, as injury of the lacrimal ducts with resulting dry eye is a possible complication.

B. Degenerative Conditions and Age-related Changes

Aneurysms, segmental thickening (varicosities), dilatations (telangiectasias), and increased tortuosity of the bulbar conjunctival vessels are not uncommon (**Ba**). They become more common with increasing age and are therefore most likely of a degenerative nature. They are generally without pathological significance but can be correlated with systemic vascular abnormalities. Occasionally, vascular abnormalities are visible in the conjunctiva over melanomas of the choroid and ciliary body or following radiation. Decreased density of the limbal vascular arcades occurs with increasing age.

The **pinguecula** (**Bb**) is a degenerative condition of the conjunctival connective tissue probably caused by chronic UV light exposure, which becomes very common with increasing age. The slightly prominent whitish or yellowish and usually triangular lesion is typically located in the nasal and more rarely in the temporal palpebral fissure at the limbus. Keratinization of the epithelium over the pinguecula (leukoplakia), calcification, or concomitant inflammation ("pingueculitis") can occasionally occur due to the permanent mechanical alteration. If it is symptomatic, treatment consists of surgical excision.

The pterygium ("winglike," **Bc** and **d**) is also a degenerative condition of the conjunctival connective tissue induced by UV light. It is relatively common, especially at an advanced age, and transition from a pinguecula to a pterygium is common. The pterygium is very well vascularized compared to the pinguecula and usually has a larger conjunctival portion (tail); it is important clinically mainly because of the corneal involvement, which is why its treatment is discussed there. Neither the pinguecula nor the pterygium undergoes malignant transformation.

Whitish calcifications in the region of the tarsal conjunctiva (calcium infarcts) become more common with increasing age. They are usually of no pathological significance and have to be removed (through a stab incision) only when there is a foreign-body sensation. Particularly in elderly and overweight persons, **prolapse of orbital fat** (**Be**) under the upper temporal conjunctiva sometimes occurs, giving the impression of a tumor. The presumed cause is dehiscence of the orbital septum. In contrast to the lipodermoid, the fat can be replaced in the orbit with a swab or similar object and the fatty tissue prolapse usually increases in size with pressure on the globe. Surgical reduction by fat resection or coagulation is required only in exceptional cases and must avoid the lacrimal ducts.

C. Various Conditions

Yellowish **discoloration** of the conjunctiva is observed in icterus, while brownish discoloration occurs, for example, in adrenocortical insufficiency (Addison disease), alkaptonuria (ochronosis), or with certain medications. Working with silver can lead to a grayish conjunctiva (argyrosis), and systemic or local exposure to iron (siderosis), gold (chrysiasis), copper (chalcosis), or arsenic leads rarely to conjunctival discoloration.

A. Malformations

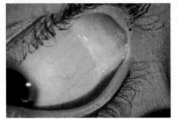

Lipodermoid, temporal

B. Degenerative Conditions and Age-related Changes

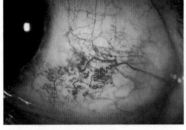

a Conjunctival vascular anomalies

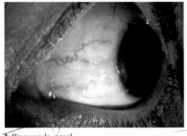

b Pinguecula, nasal

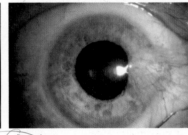

c Pterygium

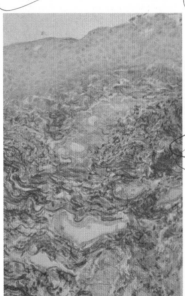

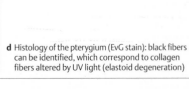

e Prolapse of orbital fat under the upper temporal conjunctiva

d Histology of the pterygium (EvG stain): black fibers can be identified, which correspond to collagen fibers altered by UV light (elastoid degeneration)

A. Various Conditions (continued)

The **circulation of the erythrocytes in the vessels of the conjunctiva** can be observed with the slit lamp. Slowing of flow ("sludging") is sometimes seen in diseases associated with increased viscosity of the blood (e. g., plasmacytoma, Waldenström disease, cryoglobulinemia) or diminished deformability of the red blood cells (e. g., sickle cell anemia).

Chemosis is the name given to edematous swelling of the conjunctiva. It occurs predominantly with conjunctival inflammation but can also be manifested separately, e. g., due to an abnormality of orbital outflow (**A**) or certain medications. Transitory conjunctival chemosis may be allergic in nature, although a causative agent often cannot be found. Drying (**xerosis**) of the conjunctiva is characterized by a dull conjunctival surface that shines little or not at all. Subsequent keratinization of the epithelial cells may occur. The xerosis usually develops as a result of long-term exposure (lagophthalmos) or major tear deficiency. Vitamin A deficiency leads rarely but typically to xerosis, which is often accentuated in the palpebral fissure region (Bitot's spots).

B. Subconjunctival Hemorrhage

Subconjunctival hemorrhage (**Ba, b**) is bleeding into the subconjunctival connective tissue.

Etiology/pathogenesis. Subconjunctival hemorrhage results from rupture or other opening of a conjunctival or episcleral blood vessel. Usually no cause can be found (idiopathic subconjunctival hemorrhage). Sometimes a prior Valsalva maneuver (e. g., coughing, straining, vomiting) is reported. Other causes of subconjunctival hemorrhage include arterial hypertension and a reduction in coagulation, e. g., due to anticoagulant medication or with leukemia. In addition, general infections associated with fever, vitamin C deficiency (scurvy), blunt or sharp eye injury, surgery on the eye, and viral conjunctivitis are possible causes.

Epidemiology. Subconjunctival hemorrhage has a high incidence. Traumatic subconjunctival hemorrhages are often observed at a younger age and idiopathic hemorrhages are often seen at a more advanced age.

Clinical features. Because of the delicate structure of the conjunctiva, even a little blood can spread diffusely in the subconjunctival connective tissue and cause diffuse erythema, which is usually of uniform intensity and conceals the blood vessels. The lower conjunctiva is affected more often than the upper. The subconjunctival hemorrhage is not very elevated, but massive hemorrhages with considerable elevation of the conjunctiva occur particularly with closed globe rupture and severe orbital injuries. The subconjunctival hemorrhage develops acutely and usually appears alarming to affected patients, though in itself it is completely harmless. Provided there are no associated (traumatic) conditions of the eye, the visual acuity is unchanged as the hemorrhage is a purely extraocular event. There is no pain.

Diagnosis. The diagnosis is made clinically and the history may assist further. When trauma is reported, injuries of the eyeball or orbit should be excluded. When an idiopathic subconjunctival hemorrhage occurs for the first time, further diagnostic measures are not usually required. In the event of recurrence, arterial hypertension and a coagulation disorder should be excluded.

Treatment. Subconjunctival hemorrhage usually does not require any treatment. Extreme forms, which lead to an abnormality of corneal moistening, can necessitate incision of the conjunctiva with drainage of the hemorrhage.

Prognosis. Spontaneous absorption of the blood takes place within a few days, and slight pigmentation persists rarely.

A. Various Conditions

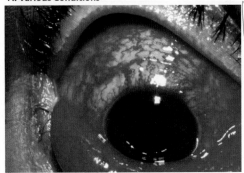

Chemosis (swelling) of the conjunctiva with massive vasodilatation in from carotid–cavernous sinus fistula

B. Subconjunctival Hemorrhage

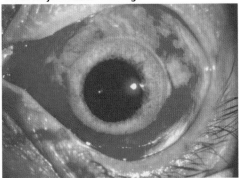

a Subconjunctival hemorrhage after contusion of the globe

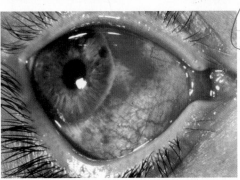

b Subconjunctival hemorrhage in viral conjunctivitis (epidemic keratoconjunctivitis)

A. Conjunctivitis

Conjunctivitis is defined as an infectious or noninfectious inflammation limited to the conjunctiva. As the conjunctiva is continuous with the epidermis at the lid margins and with the corneal epithelium at the limbus, these structures are not infrequently affected together with the conjunctiva (blepharoconjunctivitis or keratoconjunctivitis). In principle, the classical phenomena of inflammation-calor, rubor, tumor, dolor, and functio laesa (i. e., heat, redness, swelling, pain, and loss of function) -also apply to conjunctivitis; rubor ("red eye," **Aa**) has by far the greatest importance. However, the distinction of "genuine" inflammation from conjunctival hyperemia (**Ab**) is often difficult and sometimes somewhat arbitrary. Formally, primary conjunctivitis and secondary conjunctival irritation, e. g., due to intraocular processes, can be differentiated. The different forms of conjunctivitis sometimes differ considerably with regard to the etiology, clinical appearance, course, and treatment.

Etiology/pathogenesis. The conjunctiva, like the cornea, is considerably exposed to environmental influences. There is a natural defense against infection as a result of blinking, tear flow, good perfusion, plentiful local immune cells and antibacterial substances (e.g. immunoglobulins, interferons, and lysozyme of the tear film).

The varied **causes** of conjunctivitis are summarized in **Table 1** (p. 72).

The conjunctival surface is not sterile. Rather, there are normally numerous bacteria (local flora), which are usually not pathogenic. Under certain conditions, however, almost every bacterium can cause conjunctivitis. The primary factors are insufficiency of the tear film (sicca syndrome) and blinking, along with contact lenses and other factors that interfere with the natural mechanical or immunological defenses. Conjunctival infections are primarily contact infections, that is, the germs reach the eye through contaminated fingers, towels, ophthalmological equipment, etc., or close physical contact.

The allergic type I conjunctivitides (immediate type) consist particularly of allergies to pollen, grasses, and animal dander; those of delayed type usually represent reactions to chronic allergens such as eye drops, cosmetics, house dust mites, and also contact lenses. The atopic diseases that are related to the allergies (**Ac**) are probably due to hyperreactivity of the immune system. There is often an association with neurodermatitis or bronchial asthma. The causes of the common chronic "dry eye" (sicca syndrome or keratoconjunctivitis sicca) are not completely known. Hormonal disorders (androgen deficiency or an excess of female sex hormones), involution of the lacrimal glands, and also inflammatory phenomena are probably the most important in elderly patients. In children and younger adults, "dry eye" may develop as a postinflammatory event, e. g., after a viral infection. Tear deficiency states are typical of the collagenoses. They are practically inevitable in Sjögren syndrome. However, conjunctivitis sicca can also arise when tear production is adequate, or if the quality of the tear film is reduced by a mucin deficiency (loss of goblet cells) or lipid deficiency (outflow disorder of the meibomian glands, e. g., in lid margin inflammation due to rosacea). Many patients with "dry eye" report intensive work at a computer. Staring at the monitor suppresses the normal blinking reflex and thus the normal distribution of the tear film, which can then lead to sicca syndrome. Certain medications used locally or systemically can also interfere with the tear film.

A. Conjunctivitis

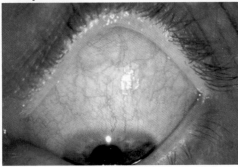

a "Red eye" as the typical sign of conjunctivitis; diffuse dilatation of the conjunctival vessels (conjunctival injection)

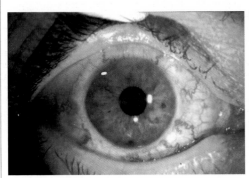

b Noninflammatory dilatation of the conjunctival vessels (hyperemia) in orbital outflow disorder (carotid–cavernous sinus fistula); in contrast to the inflammatory erythema, the vasodilatation is more marked but is also confined to fewer vessels

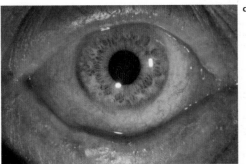

c Atopic conjunctivitis with thickening of the lid margin and erythema of the skin of the lid

Table 1 Causes and treatment of conjunctivitis

Cause		Treatment
Bacteria	• Staphylococcus aureus Staphylococcus epidermidis Streptococcus pneumoniae Haemophilus influenzae	• Astringent, antiseptic, or antibiotic eye drops (aminoglycosides or gyrase inhibitors); débridement of the lid margins and lacrimal ducts
	• Neisseria gonorrhoeae (gonoblennorrhea))	• Local and systemic antibiotic (penicillin), protection of the unaffected eye
	• Chlamydia trachomatis serotypes A–C (trachoma) Chlamydia trachomatis serotypes D–K ("swimming pool conjunctivitis")	• Tetracycline (not in children) or erythromycin eye drops, possibly systemic treatment and treatment of the opposite eye
	• Other	
Viruses	• Herpes simplex virus (HSV) Varicella zoster virus (VZV)	• Virustatic agents only exceptionally, usually spontaneous healing
	• Adenovirus types 8 and 19 (epidemic keratoconjunctivitis)	• Symptomatic measures (tear substitute), prevention of spread (hygiene)
	• Molluscum contagiosum near to the lid margin	• Excision of molluscum contagiosum
	• Measles, rubella, and mumps virus	• None required
	• Others	
Fungi	• Especially Candida albicans (with immunosuppression)	• Antimycotic eye drops
Parasites	• E. g., onchocerciasis or Loa loa	• Antiparasitic medications, surgical removal of subconjunctival worms
Allergies and atopic diseases		• Avoidance of allergen; local mast cell stabilizers, antihistamines, anti-inflammatories (corticosteroids), in certain cases cyclosporine eye drops, tear substitute, rarely systemic immunosuppression
Contact lens-induced giant papilla conjunctivitis		• Avoidance of contact lenses

Cause		Treatment
Tear film insufficiency (sicca syndrome)		• Tear substitute, cyclosporine eye drops, débridement of the lid margins; in severe cases occlusion of the lacrimal punctum, in future possibly local hormone therapy (androgens)
Immunological diseases	• Ocular pemphigoid Paraneoplastic pemphigoid Endocrine orbitopathy Graft-versus-host reaction after bone marrow transplantation Stevens–Johnson syndrome	• Systemic immunosuppression, tear substitute (without preservatives), rarely surgical measures, discontinuation of causative medications
Vasculitides	• Wegener granulomatosis Primary chronic polyarthritis Kawasaki syndrome	• Treatment of the underlying disease, symptomatic measures in the eye
Metabolic disorders	• Gout Plasminogen deficiency (conjunctivitis lignosa)	• Treatment of the underlying disease, symptomatic measures in the eye
Mechanical effects	• Foreign bodies Disorder of differentiation of the limbus epithelium (super-ior limbic keratoconjunctivitis) Trichiasis (entropion)	• (Surgical) Elimination of the cause, conjunctival resection in superior limbic keratoconjunctivitis
Toxic chemical and thermal effects	• Corrosive injuries Burns	• Acute dilution of the causative agent or cooling; treatment and prevention of secondary complications
Reaction to medications	• Stevens–Johnson syndrome Lyell syndrome Toxic conjunctivitis, e. g., in reaction to aspirin or antibiotics	• Avoidance of the causative medication; treatment and prevention of secondary complications (e. g., prevention of adhe-sions (symblephara)
Exposure	• Nonclosing eyelids (lagophthalmos) Lid deformity (ectropion)	• Tear substitute; surgical reduction of the palpebral fissure, surgical correction of the lid deformity
Asthenopia	• Latent hyperopia • Heterophoria	• Optic correction • Prism glasses, squint operation

A. Conjunctivitis (continued)

Epidemiology. Conjunctivitis is the most frequent disease of the eyes overall. About 10% of all neonates develop conjunctivitis for various reasons (**A, Table 1**). It has been estimated that about 1–3% of all wearers of contact lenses are affected with giant papillary conjunctivitis. Conjunctival inflammation occurs at every age, but certain forms are found more often in certain age groups. For instance, vernal keratoconjunctivitis is primarily a disease of children, while atopic keratoconjunctivitis and allergic conjunctivitis are typically diseases of adolescents and young adults. The cicatricial conjunctivitides represent diseases of more advanced age.

Infectious conjunctivitis affects both sexes with roughly the same incidence. Conjunctivitis due to chemical or mechanical causes and vernal keratoconjunctivitis are markedly more common in males, while conjunctivitis sicca occurs much more often in females.

Clinical features. With the exception of injury, conjunctivitis usually develops bilaterally, though the degree of severity is often asymmetrical. It is typical of epidemic keratoconjunctivitis that the second eye is usually affected less than the first, as a result of antibody production.

Symptoms and signs in conjunctivitis:

- **Foreign body sensation** ("a feeling like sand in the eyes").
- **"Red eye"** (see p. 71, **Aa**). Normally the eye is white because the conjunctival and episcleral vessels are not visible or are barely visible against the white background of the sclera. The white eye turns into a "red eye" only through dilatation of the epibulbar vessels. The (historical) distinction between conjunctival injection (more superficial) and ciliary injection (deeper and more pronounced at the limbus) is often not helpful in routine clinical practice as there are often varied presentations.

  In conjunctivitis the entire conjunctiva is usually reddened. Toxic conjunctival irritation prefers the lower parts of the conjunctiva. Superior limbic keratoconjunctivitis (**Aa**), as the name suggests, is limited to the upper margin of the cornea. In conjunctivitis sicca and conjunctivitis due to *Chlamydia*, the redness is often only slight or not apparent at all.

- **Epiphora (abnormal overflow of tears).** Tearing is an expression of reflexly increased tear production, and is more rarely an outflow disorder (due to swelling). It is found typically in conditions of the cornea but can also occur in conjunctivitis, particularly epidemic **keratoconjunctivitis**.
- **Secretion from the conjunctival sac.** This secretion is usually yellowish and creamy purulent in bacterial conjunctivitis (**Ab**), while it is usually watery and clear in viral conjunctivitis. In allergic and atopic conjunctivitis and in conjunctivitis due to *Chlamydia*, the secretions are usually viscous and mucoid (**Ac**).
- **Adhesion of the lids.** This is usually found in the mornings as the mucus or secretion dries during the night. Adhesion of the lids is very typical of bacterial conjunctival infections.
- **Itching.** Most forms of conjunctivitis are not itchy. However, itching is typical of allergic and atopic conjunctivitis, which also include contact lens-induced giant papillary conjunctivitis. Parasitic conjunctival infections are also usually associated with severe itching.

A. Conjunctivitis

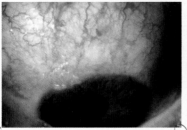

a Superior limbic keratoconjunctivitis: redness of the upper conjunctiva with whitish epithelial change at the limbus

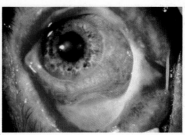

b Purulent secretion as evidence of bacterial conjunctivitis

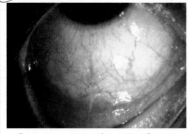

c Allergic conjunctivitis with secretion of viscous mucus

Table 1 Causes, time of appearance, and incidence of neonatal conjunctivitis

Disease/cause	Time of appearance	Incidence
Toxic irritation due to Credé prophylaxis (1% silver nitrate)	A few hours after application of drops	Has become rare due to antibiotic prophylaxis today
Gonoblennorhea/intrapartum infection with Neisseria gonorrhoeae	1 – 4 days postpartum	Has become very rare because of prophylaxis
Other intrapartum infection with bacteria (e.g., Streptococcus pneumoniae, Haemophilus influenzae, staphylococci, Pseudomonas aeruginosa, etc.)	4 – 6 days postpartum	Not rare
Intrapartum infection with herpes simplex virus (HSV)	5 – 7 days postpartum	Not rare
Intrapartum infection with Chlamydia trachomatis	4 – 15 (usually 7 – 10) days postpartum	Most frequent cause of neonatal conjunctivitis

A. Conjunctivitis (continued)

Clinical features (continued). Other symptoms and signs:

- **Pain.** Conjunctivitis is usually only slightly painful or not painful. Pain is reported especially when the cornea is also involved, as in epidemic keratoconjunctivitis and in conjunctivitis sicca, despite the fact that the clinical signs are often rather slight.

- **Photophobia.** Photophobia is not a typical symptom of most conjunctivitides but often occurs in epidemic keratoconjunctivitis.

- **Swelling of the conjunctiva (chemosis).** This is observed particularly in adenoviral epidemic keratoconjunctivitis but is also highly typical of allergic and parasitic conjunctivitis. Chemosis of the conjunctiva is also found very often in florid endocrine orbitopathy.

- **Subconjunctival hemorrhage.** This develops preferentially in viral conjunctivitis, especially epidemic keratoconjunctivitis, more rarely in bacterial conjunctivitis.

- **Follicle production (Aa).** Viral and chlamydial and also medication-induced conjunctivitis leads to the formation of nodules (follicles) that are visible with the slit lamp. They correspond to accumulations of lymphocytes and occur particularly in the region of the fornices (follicular conjunctivitis). Trachoma was given the name of "Egyptian granular disease" because of the very large granular follicles and because of the introduction of the disease to Western Europe as a result of the North African expedition of Napoleon I at the end of the 18th century. Because the function of their immune system is still limited, infants do not develop follicular conjunctivitis.

- **Papilla formation (Ab).** In the region of the lids, the conjunctiva is fixed relatively firmly to the tarsus by strands of connective tissue. The tarsal conjunctiva can therefore swell only very little compared to the bulbar conjunctiva. In the case of swelling, the fixing connective tissue strands can lead to contractions, so that "warts" (papillae) develop that have a vessel at their center (papillary conjunctivitis). These papillae are usually small but can become very big, especially in vernal keratoconjunctivitis and allergic reactions to mainly but not exclusively soft contact lenses (giant papillary conjunctivitis), and produce a cobblestone-like pattern.

- **Membrane production (Ac).** Genuine membranes can be distinguished from pseudomembranes. The former lead to bleeding on removal, while the latter do not. Classically, diphtheria, which rarely occurs today, leads to genuine conjunctival membranes. However, membranes, like pseudomembranes, can also occur in other bacterial and viral conjunctival infections (pseudomembranous conjunctivitis). Pseudomembranes are also found in allergic or toxic (medication-induced) conjunctivitis. A special form of membrane formation is found in conjunctivitis lignosa ("woody conjunctivitis"), in which the conjunctival deposits usually have a tough consistency (Ad).

- **Marked redness and swelling of caruncle and plica semilunaris (Ae).** This is particularly characteristic of epidemic keratoconjunctivitis but is also often observed in florid endocrine orbitopathy.

- **Adhesions (symblephara, Af).** Adhesions of the tarsal and bulbar conjunctiva are more frequent in the region of the lower conjunctival sac than in the upper. They are practically inevitable with chronic cicatricial conjunctivitis (ocular and medication-induced pemphigoid) and advanced trachoma, commonly found with atopic conjunctivitis, and occasionally occur following pseudomembranous conjunctivitis of various origins and in dry eye. Scleroderma and ichthyosis are often associated with conjunctival adhesions. When the symblephara are more severe, there is a reduction in eye motility.

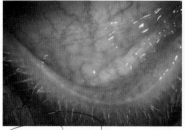

a Follicular conjunctivitis

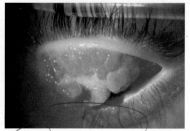

b Papillary conjunctivitis: typical "cobblestones" in the tarsal conjunctiva in vernal conjunctivitis

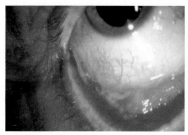

c Membrane formation in epidemic keratoconjunctivitis

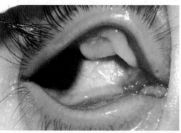

d Thick "woody" membrane in keratoconjunctivitis lignosa (plasminogen deficiency)

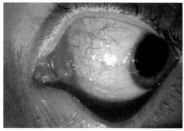

e Marked erythema of the caruncle in epidemic keratoconjunctivitis

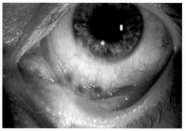

f Symblepharon (adhesion of bulbar and tarsal conjunctiva) in atopic keratoconjunctivitis

A. Conjunctivitis (continued)

Clinical features (continued). Other symptoms and signs:

- **Lid margin parallel conjunctival folds (LIP-COF).** Characteristic of conjunctivitis sicca.
- **Lid conditions.** A large number of cases of conjunctivitis lead to accompanying redness and swelling of the lids. The latter is typical of epidemic keratoconjunctivitis and particularly of gonococcal conjunctivitis (gonoblennorrhea). The swelling can give the impression of a drooping upper lid (pseudoptosis). Chronic allergic conjunctivitis is not infrequently associated with redness and scaling of the periorbital lid skin (allergic contact eczema or atopic dermatitis).
- **Associated corneal conditions.** In epidemic keratoconjunctivitis, superficial roundish opacities of the cornea occur usually 5–15 days after the acute manifestation (**Aa**). These opacities, known as nummules, are an expression of an antigen-antibody reaction and indicate that there is no or only a slight risk of contagion. Peripheral subepithelial corneal infiltrates and superficial vascular growth into the peripheral cornea (pannus) are sometimes found in the course of chlamydial conjunctivitis. Vernal keratoconjunctivitis and atopic keratoconjunctivitis in their tarsal papillary forms are occasionally associated with shieldlike corneal opacities and in their limbic forms with whitish opacities at the margin of the cornea. These so-called Trantas dots (**Ab**) can rarely also be observed in contact lens-associated giant papillary conjunctivitis. In some marked forms of "dry eye" threads of mucus are found on the cornea (filiform keratitis). Chronic rosacea conjunctivitis is often associated with peripheral corneal vascularization. Chronic cicatricial conjunctivitis such as ocular pemphigoid or linear IgA dermatosis (**Ac**) often leads to considerable vascular proliferation and diffuse corneal opacity. *Neisseria gonorrhoeae* is extremely dangerous as it can easily penetrate the intact cornea, and lead to corneal perforation. Blindness from gonorrheal conjunctivitis was therefore very common until the end of the 19th century.
- **Swelling of regional lymph nodes.** The lymphatic vessels of the conjunctiva drain into the preauricular and submandibular lymph nodes. Swelling of the lymph nodes is typical of epidemic keratoconjunctivitis, but sometimes also occurs in chlamydial and some other bacterial conjunctivitides. Parinaud oculoglandular syndrome is an etiologically diverse but usually bacterial and granulomatous unilateral conjunctivitis with associated swelling of the regional lymph nodes.
- **General symptoms.** Epidemic keratoconjunctivitis is occasionally associated with general (flulike) symptoms, while conjunctivitis of other causation is not commonly associated with systemic symptoms.
- **Intraocular conditions.** Pure conjunctivitis is almost never associated with intraocular inflammation, alteration of the pupil, or change in ocular pressure. Chronic cicatricial conjunctivitis is an exception, in which glaucoma can occur because of displacement of the episcleral veins. Rarely, inflammatory exudates on the corneal endothelium are found in epidemic keratoconjunctivitis. Visual acuity is usually not affected by conjunctivitis or, if it is, acuity is reduced only slightly (by the epiphora) unless secondary corneal complications have developed. A reduction in vision, an irregular pupil, or increased ocular pressure in combination with a "red eye" argue against the diagnosis of primary conjunctivitis.

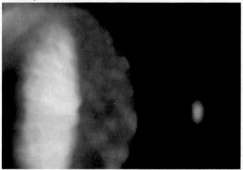

a Roundish superficial corneal opacities (nummules) in epidemic keratoconjunctivitis

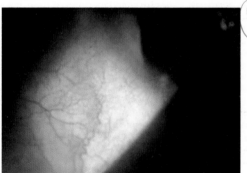

b Whitish infiltrates (Trantas dots) in vernal keratoconjunctivitis

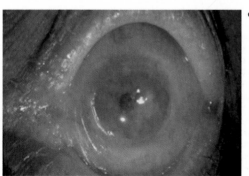

c Corneal opacities in chronic cicatricial conjunctivitis (linear IgA dermatosis)

A. Conjunctivitis (continued)

Diagnosis. Diagnosis begins with the **history**. The course (acute/chronic) gives information about the cause. The season also provides evidence for the origin of the conjunctivitis. For instance, allergic rhinoconjunctivitis is manifested in the spring from increased pollen, while vernal keratoconjunctivitis is exacerbated primarily in spring until fall ("spring catarrh"). Fall and winter are the periods of predilection for epidemic keratoconjunctivitis. Known allergies such as hay fever or asthma point to allergic or atopic conjunctivitis and certain activities suggest possible foreign body-induced conjunctivitis. Giant papillary conjunctivitis usually develops about ten months after starting to wear contact lenses. If associated with swimming, the conjunctivitis might be chlamydial ("swimming-pool conjunctivitis"). Certain systemic diseases such as rheumatoid arthritis, Sjögren syndrome, Wegener granulomatosis, Kawasaki syndrome, or graft-versus-host (GVH) reaction, may have associated conjunctivitis. However, the conjunctivitis sometimes precedes the systemic manifestations. In the case of infectious conjunctivitis, the time of inoculation is often unknown. An exception is the highly infectious epidemic keratoconjunctivitis, which has an incubation period of about 5–10 days. The history often reveals that relatives or friends have had a "red eye" or there has been a visit to an eye specialist (infection from another patient or measurement of ocular pressure with contaminated instruments). In bacterial conjunctivitis, the second eye is usually affected 2–3 days after the first. Neonatal conjunctivitis has various causes, which can be suspected from the time at which they occur (see p. 75, **Table 1**). Following the history, the diagnosis is made from the **symptoms** and the **clinical appearance**. This often allows etiological classification of the conjunctivitis. The entire conjunctival sac should always be inspected (single and if necessary double eversion). Other investigations include:

- Swab for microbiological examination (smear or bacterial culture).
- Swab for detection of molecular genetic pathogens (bacteria or viruses) by the polymerase chain reaction (PCR).
- Smear of a superficial scrape of the conjunctiva. Besides conjunctival epithelial cells, neutrophil granulocytes are found particularly in bacterial and mycotic conjunctivitis, mainly lymphocytes in viral conjunctivitis, and a mixed picture of neutrophils and lymphocytes in chlamydial infections, sometimes with intracytoplasmic inclusion bodies in the epithelial cells. Eosinophilic and sometimes basophilic granulocytes are usually found in allergic, atopic, and giant papillary conjunctivitis.
- Measurement of tear secretion using strips of filter paper (Schirmer's test I, II) and measurement of tear quality by determining the tear film break-up time.
- Morphological diagnosis using impression cytology or conjunctival biopsy is employed especially to confirm the diagnosis of cicatricial conjunctivitis (ocular pemphigoid) or to exclude a diffuse (pagetoid) tumor imitating conjunctivitis. In massive sicca syndrome and vitamin A deficiency, keratinization of the epithelium can often be identified.
- Allergy testing.
- Measurement of autoantibodies, e.g., when Wegener disease, lupus erythematosus, or Sjögren syndrome is suspected.
- **Consultation with other specialists.** When conjunctivitis is suspected to be due to a systemic disease, consultation may be necessary. Sjögren syndrome is usually confirmed by biopsy of the oral mucosa. Chronic cicatricial conjunctivitis such as ocular pemphigoid, atopic diseases, and some allergies require collaboration with a dermatologist.

Differential diagnosis. The symptom of "red eye" is not diagnostic of conjunctivitis. The differential diagnosis must therefore consider all diseases that can be associated with secondary reddening of the conjunctiva. These include, in particular, keratitis, anterior uveitis (iritis or iridocyclitis), and acute narrow-angle glaucoma, but previous surgery, an immunological corneal graft reaction, neovascular diseases, disorders of orbital outflow (e.g., carotid-cavernous sinus fistula), or tumors should also be considered. It is often difficult to distinguish conjunctivitis from episcleritis, which is usually unilateral and has few symptoms. The latter is usually less diffuse or more circumscribed and is associated with dilatation of deeper vessels. The distinction is often made by manual displacement of the conjunctiva against the sclera (if the dilated vessels can be displaced easily, they are more likely to be in the conjunctiva than in the episclera) or local application of a sympathomimetic drop, which leads to constriction of the superficial (conjunctival) but less of the deeper (episcleral) vessels. It is often difficult clinically to distinguish hyperemia of the conjunctiva, such as that which occurs in chronic alcoholism, in certain metabolic disorders, or after prolonged use of various medications, from conjunctivitis.

Treatment. Treatment is guided by the (suspected) cause of the conjunctivitis (see p. 72, **Table 1**). The majority of cases of conjunctivitis heal fully without treatment. Since complications of conjunctivitis occur only rarely, there is usually a risk of overtreatment rather than undertreatment. In general, local antibiotics and corticosteroids should be used selectively because of their side-effects (risk of developing antibiotic resistance and allergies; cost in the case of antibiotics, and risk of inducing or exacerbating a herpetic, bacterial, or mycotic infection; glaucoma and cataract with more prolonged use of corticosteroids). In many cases, symptomatic measures (cleansing of the conjunctival sac and lid margins with tap water) are sufficient. "Household remedies" such as chamomile solutions should be avoided as these increase rather than improve the conjunctival irritation. Antiseptic or astringent eye drops often shorten or alleviate the symptoms, the latter by constricting the vessels ("whiteners"). In bacterial conjunctivitis, examination of the cornea is necessary so that any ulceration can be identified promptly. Use of an eye patch increases the temperature over the eye and thus may promote bacterial growth.

Prognosis. The prognosis in most types of conjunctivitis is generally very good. Complete healing usually occurs within a few days, though epidemic keratoconjunctivitis can cause symptoms for several weeks or even months because of the nummular corneal infiltrates or "dry eye". Loss of function due to corneal complications occurs particularly in the chronic forms such as atopic conjunctivitis, in vernal keratoconjunctivitis, and above all in cicatricial forms of conjunctivitis. Since infectious (bacterial or viral) conjunctivitis usually does not lead to permanent immunity, recurrences are possible. Repeated episodes are characteristic of the allergic and atopic types of conjunctivitis. Sicca syndrome occasionally resolves spontaneously, especially when it is of a postinfectious nature. However, it often persists indefinitely.

Particular caution is indicated with neonatal bacterial conjunctivitis since systemic complications such as sepsis, orbital cellulitis, or meningitis are possible because of the physiological immune incompetence.

A. Tumors

Numerous benign and malignant tumors occur in the conjunctiva, but the spectrum is much narrower than in the lids, for example. Conjunctival neoplasms are predominantly of epithelial and melanocytic origin. In addition, there are the much rarer lymphatic, vascular, neurogenic, myogenic, and metastatic neoplasms. Not a few tumors of the conjunctiva are of a degenerative or reactive nature. Some are congenital hamartomas (= tumors of cells from that site) or choristomas (= tumors with parts that do not normally occur at that site). Overall, the bulbar conjunctiva is affected much more often by tumors than the tarsal conjunctiva. Most conjunctival neoplasms are noticed because of their visibility. Tumors growing on the cornea can lead to a reduction in vision by inducing astigmatism or altering the tear film. Very large neoplasms can sometimes interfere with globe motility. Tumors of the tarsal conjunctiva sometimes displace the lacrimal punctum so that epiphora occurs.

Benign tumors. Squamous epithelial papillomas often have a cauliflower-like surface (**Aa**). Numerous vessels sprouting within the subepithelial connective tissue are typical. The tumors are broad-based (sessile) or narrow-based (pedunculated). They are often caused by human papilloma viruses (HPVs), especially in younger persons. Epithelial dysplasia and carcinoma in situ, which should be regarded as precancerous, are intraepithelial in location and usually not prominent. A whitish color, termed leukoplakia (**Ab**), is often seen as an expression of superficial keratinization (leukoplakia tends to suggest a benign lesion but can also occur in malignant epithelial processes).

The commonest melanocytic conjunctival tumor is the nevus (**Ac**). This is considered to be a (congenital) hamartoma and arises from proliferation of melanocytes in the region of the basal epithelium (junctional nevus). Through "dripping" and "maturation" of the melanocytes, the nevus subsequently involves the subepithelial connective tissue (compound nevus, ultimately subepithelial nevus). Conjunctival nevi, which are often only slightly pigmented, are found in children and adolescents in the bulbar conjunctiva. In times of hormonal change (such as puberty), these nevi can enlarge and change color. "Nevi" developing at an advanced age or on the tarsal conjunctiva are usually malignant melanomas. On slit-lamp examination and histology, small cysts are often seen within the nevi (**Ad**).

At an advanced age, flat areas of pigmentation are sometimes found, which are known as acquired epithelial melanosis (**Ae**). Histologically, a benign type can be distinguished from a type tending to malignant degeneration (= premelanoma). Congenital conjunctival choristomas (limbal dermoid and lipodermoid) and the tumorlike conditions due to degeneration of the conjunctival connective tissue (pinguecula and pterygium) have already been mentioned. Conjunctival cysts can usually be transilluminated. Reactive tumors include foreign-body granuloma (e. g., as a reaction to suture material used in ocular muscle surgery, **Af**) and pyogenic granuloma (**Ag**). Pyogenic granulomas correspond histologically to highly vascular granulation tissue, which gives the often rapidly growing tumor a reddish color. They usually develop after an operation or a (trivial) injury; more often they occur with a chalazion. Lymphangiomas often have bleeding into the tumor. Fibromas, neurofibromas, neurinomas, lipomas, leiomyomas, hemangiomas, and benign lymphatic tumors are rarities in the conjunctiva.

The caruncle has a different morphological structure from the conjunctiva. It is only here that skin appendages such as hairs and sebaceous glands are found. This explains why the range of tumors at the caruncle differs from that of the remainder of the conjunctiva. Thus, the usually reddish or brownish oncocytoma (**Ah**), which probably arises from degeneration of glandular cells, occurs almost only in the caruncle.

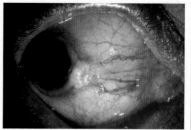

a Papilloma of the conjunctiva

b Leukoplakia ("white spot") of the conjunctiva

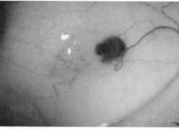

c Nonpigmented nevus of the conjunctiva with focal pigmentation; the typical clear cysts can just be seen

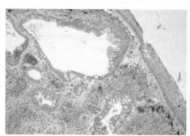

d Histology of an excised conjunctival nevus

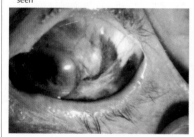

e Primary acquired melanosis of the conjunctiva

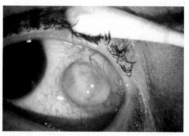

f Foreign body granuloma

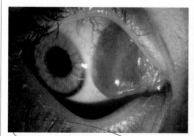

g Pyogenic granuloma of the conjunctiva

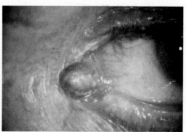

h Oncocytoma of the caruncle

A. Tumors (continued)

Malignant tumors. Malignant tumors are rare in the conjunctiva. Conjunctival squamous cell carcinoma, which can develop from a papilloma or epithelial dysplasia, occurs at a later age and usually has a glassy gelatinous appearance (**Aa**). Particularly in the so-called mucoepidermoid variant, it can penetrate the sclera along preformed channels (emissaries) and extend into the inside of the eye.

Malignant melanomas of the conjunctiva (**Ab**) arise predominantly from acquired epithelial melanosis, more rarely from normal conjunctiva (de novo) or from a nevus. These tumors are usually not quite black but rather brownish and are situated preferentially in the bulbar conjunctiva. Middle-aged and elderly people are affected. Conjunctival malignant melanomas in childhood are extremely rare. Malignant non-Hodgkin lymphoma (NHL) of the conjunctiva (**Ac**) usually has a characteristic salmon-yellow color. It is one of the so-called MALT (mucosa-associated lymphoid tissue) lymphomas, which are characterized by persistence for years without significant progression. In AIDS, Kaposi sarcoma can occur on the conjunctiva. Malignant neoplasms of the lids such as basal cell carcinoma, squamous cell carcinoma, and sebaceous gland carcinoma can extend to the conjunctiva by direct growth. Primary intraocular tumors, usually choroid malignant melanoma, sometimes grow through the sclera and may then appear to be conjunctival tumors (**Ad**). Metastases from tumors distant from the eye are very unusual in the conjunctiva but are possible (**Ae**). The primary tumors are mainly lung cancer, breast cancer, and cutaneous malignant melanoma.

Diagnosis. The diagnosis is usually made from the clinical appearance, the history (rate of growth), and, as the range of tumors differs at different ages, from the age of the patient. By means of transillumination (diaphanoscopy) and high-resolution ultrasound (ultrasonic biomicroscopy), a distinction can be made between a solid and a cystic neoplasm. In case of doubt, a biopsy of the conjunctiva can be performed readily to allow histological tumor diagnosis.

Differential diagnosis. The differential diagnosis includes inflammatory conditions in particular. For instance, nodular scleritis can look like a conjunctival tumor. Conversely, it is also possible for a tumor such as a (pagetoid) sebaceous gland carcinoma growing diffusely in the conjunctival epithelium to look like inflammation ("masquerade syndrome"). Foreign bodies that have penetrated the conjunctiva and have become secondarily encapsulated can occasionally mimic a tumor.

With malignant conjunctival tumors capable of metastasis, such as squamous cell carcinoma and in particular malignant melanoma, palpation and possibly ultrasound examination of the regional, preauricular, and submandibular lymph nodes should not be omitted. Conjunctival melanoma and conjunctival NHL in particular require staging by an internist to exclude systemic manifestation.

Treatment. Tumors without suspected metastasis can be observed ("watchful waiting"). A photographic record is useful in monitoring the course. Troublesome tumors and those suspected of malignancy should be excised completely (excisional biopsy). This can usually be done relatively easily under local anesthesia. Sometimes, only a small piece is taken from large tumors (incisional biopsy) in order to obtain a diagnosis initially. In the case of squamous cell carcinoma and malignant melanoma, some healthy tissue must also be removed from the margins of the tumor in order to remove any residual tumor cells.

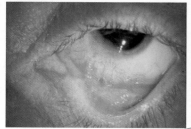

a Squamous cell carcinoma of the conjunctiva

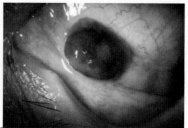

b Malignant melanoma of the conjunctiva, arising from primary acquired melanosis

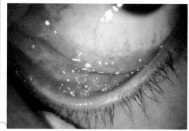

c Non-Hodgkin lymphoma (NHL) of the conjunctiva with typical salmon-colored appearance

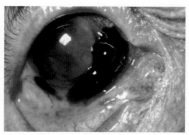

d Malignant melanoma of the choroid, growing outward through the sclera, mimics primary conjunctival melanoma

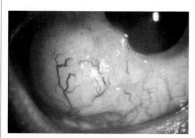

e Conjunctival metastasis from a squamous cell carcinoma

A. Tumors (continued)

Treatment (continued). Adjuvant cryotherapy or adjuvant radiotherapy can sometimes be required. Apart from NHL of the conjunctiva, radiotherapy does not play an important part in the primary treatment of conjunctival neoplasms. Conditions situated within the epithelium that can change into an invasive tumor (e.g., carcinoma in situ and primary acquired melanosis) are accessible to cytostatic treatment with mitomycin C drops (0.02 %). The conjunctival defect remaining after tumor excision usually closes spontaneously. It should be ensured that adhesion of the bulbar and tarsal conjunctiva (symblepharon) does not occur. The conjunctival sac must sometimes be wiped repeatedly or an Illig shell must be inserted. Very large conjunctival defects require reconstructive treatment in the form of an oral mucosa graft, an amniotic membrane graft, or a conjunctival graft from the other eye.

When malignant conjunctival tumors have penetrated into the orbit, the entire orbital contents usually have to be removed (exenteration of the orbit). Metastasis from squamous cell carcinoma and malignant melanoma of the conjunctiva is usually lymphatogenous at first. Surgical clearance of the regional lymph nodes (neck dissection) can therefore still be curative. At the stage of hematogenous distant metastasis, particularly with conjunctival melanoma, all the currently available therapies can at best increase life expectancy but cannot produce cure.

Prognosis. The prognosis of conjunctival tumors is generally very good. However, recurrences of the malignant neoplasms and even of the biologically benign pterygium are frequent. A fatal outcome is very rare with squamous cell carcinoma. In contrast, the mortality of conjunctival NHL is about 5–10 %, and is about 20–30 % in conjunctival melanoma, where the prognosis depends mainly on the location and thickness of the tumor. For the very unusual conjunctival metastasis, survival is usually only a few months.

B. Injuries

Injuries of the conjunctiva affecting mainly children and young men are very frequent. They include subconjunctival hemorrhage, superficial abrasions, foreign bodies, and lacerations. Foreign bodies penetrate the conjunctiva in the course of occupational or leisure activities. They usually consist of metal, glass (including broken glasses), sand, or organic material (wood, insects). Removing them from the lower conjunctival sac with a cotton tipped applicator or tweezers is usually unproblematic. If they are in the upper conjunctival sac, irrigation of the conjunctival sac and single or double eversion of the upper lid is occasionally required for their removal (**Ba** and **b**). Scratches on the cornea often provide indirect evidence of a subtarsal foreign body. Rarely, foreign bodies that are not removed are incorporated into the conjunctiva or subconjunctival connective tissue (**Bc–f**). Lacerations of the conjunctiva occur due to sharp and less often due to blunt injuries (**Bg**). Smaller tears do not require any treatment. Larger tears are usually sutured, especially when the more deeply located connective tissue of Tenon's capsule is also involved. Traumatic defects of conjunctival substance occur very rarely. Corrosive injuries (**Bh**) will be discussed in Chapter 8, "Cornea". Subconjunctival air (emphysema) can occur with fractures of the paranasal cavities.

Apart from the sometimes harmful corrosive injuries, conjunctival injuries very rarely cause persistent functional damage. However, in the case of lacerations and massive subconjunctival bleeding, involvement of the globe (e.g., in the form of a scleral perforation or an intraocular foreign body) should be ruled out. In case of doubt, inspection of the sclera and funduscopy with the pupil dilated are indicated.

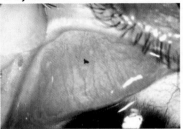

a Subtarsal foreign body after simple lid eversion

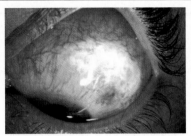

b Superficial splash of paint on the conjunctiva

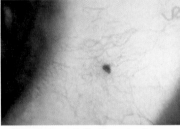

c Foreign body penetrating the conjunctiva (subconjunctival)

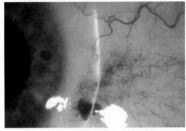

d Black gunpowder penetrating the conjunctiva

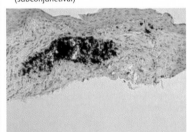

e Black gunpowder penetrating the conjunctiva; histology following conjunctival excision

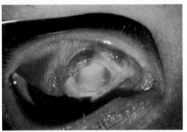

f "Forgotten" contact lens scarred onto the upper tarsus

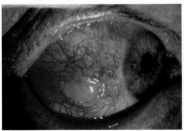

g Tear of the conjunctiva with incipient infection; injury from a cat's paw

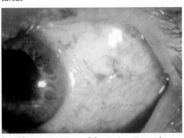

h Mild corrosion injury of the conjunctiva with disrupted vessels

A. Malformations and Anomalies

Complete **absence of the cornea** is a very rare condition and is usually associated with other anomalies of the eye. In **microcornea** the corneal diameter in adults is >10 mm. In megalocornea the corneal diameter is >13 mm. Microcornea and megalocornea can be associated with systemic malformations and generalized diseases. Tumors of the cornea are rare and are often only secondary to conjunctival tumors. The commonest tumor of the cornea is the **epibulbar dermoid** situated at the limbus. The tumor occurs as part of **Goldenhar syndrome** (facioauriculovertebral syndrome) (**A**). This is a noninherited embryogenetic malformation of the structures of the first branchial arch of unknown cause. About two-thirds are male. The incidence is 1 : 3000 births. The unilateral malformation is associated with involvement of the face and neck region. Additional findings are ocular colobomas, hypoplasia of the auricle, preauricular appendages, strabismus, and spinal malformations. The limbal dermoid should be excised if there is a risk of amblyopia, astigmatism, or exposure keratitis. Congenital conditions of the cornea associated with **glaucoma** are dealt with in Chapter 12.

B. Corneal Degeneration

Corneal degeneration is a nonhereditary, secondary, progressive change in association with age and ocular and systemic diseases.

C. Age-related Degenerative Conditions

Age-related degenerative conditions often do not require treatment. **Arcus senilis** (**C**) is seen in nearly all persons over 80 years, but when it occurs in young persons a disorder of lipid metabolism must be considered. Clinically there is a bilateral, ring-shaped, whitish, peripheral stromal opacity with a clear gap between it and the limbus. The **Vogt limbus band** is a half-moon shaped, whitish, limbally located opacity in the region of the lid fissure. **Crocodile shagreen** are gray-white polygonal opacities in the anterior or posterior stroma, which are separated by clear gaps. Peripherally located collagen formations of the endothelial cells are called **Hassall-Henle bodies**, and when centrally located are called **cornea guttata**. They can be the first stage of Fuchs endothelial dystrophy.

D. Central Degenerations

Lipid keratopathy occurs after corneal trauma, herpes simplex, or herpes zoster keratitis (secondary form) and shows homogenous, large yellow-white vascularized stromal deposits. The primary form is avascular. **Band keratopathy** (**Da**) arises from deposition of calcium in the region of the lid fissure at the level of Bowman's membrane in association with chronic eye diseases (e. g., chronic iridocyclitis, phthisis, or hypercalcemia). A possible therapy is application of EDTA plus abrasion. **Nodular Salzmann degeneration** (**Db**) occurs after chronic keratitis. Clinically there are circular, subepithelial, whitish stromal nodules of the middle of the corneal periphery.

E. Peripheral Degeneration

In staphylococcal-induced **marginal keratitis** (**Ea**), subepithelial infiltrates are apparent in the 2-, 4-, 8-, and 10-o'clock positions, which are separated from the limbus by a clear gap. There is a good response to treatment with local steroids. **Terrien's marginal degeneration** (**Eb**) is a progressive, bilateral, usually asymptomatic thinning of the corneal stroma, which begins in the superior cornea; the origin is unclear and 75 % of cases occur in men. Perforation occurs in up to 15 % of cases. **Mooren's ulcer** is an autoimmune process that in elderly patients leads to unilateral, painful infiltration at the limbus that extends circularly and centrally. **Dellen** are round epithelial defects and corneal thinning associated with local corneal dehydration.

A. Malformations and Anomalies

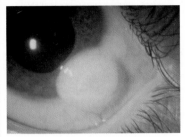

Epidermoid in Goldenhar syndrome

C. Age-related Degeneration

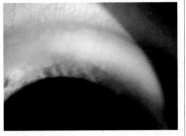

Arcus senilis

D. Central Degenerations

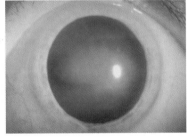

a Band keratopathy

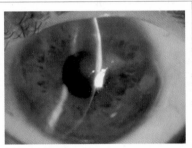

b Salzmann degeneration

E. Peripheral Degeneration

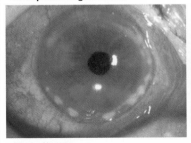

a Marginal keratitis

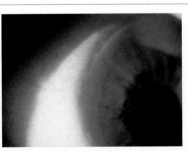

b Terrien marginal degeneration

A. Degeneration in Systemic Diseases

Epithelial keratitis, inflammation, and vascularization of the inferior cornea with subepithelial infiltrates and corneal thinning occur in 5 % of **rosacea** (**Aa**). This predominantly affects female patients between 30 and 40 years of age. Dermatological signs include papules, pustules, telangiectasias, and hypertrophic sebaceous glands. Treatment often includes local steroids and systemic tetracyclines. Keratitis can also occur in the **collagenoses**. In **rheumatoid arthritis** (**Ab**) there can be peripheral corneal alterations such as sclerosing keratitis, limbal corneal ulceration, and thinning, which typically occur with "burnt-out" joint disease and require systemic immunosuppression.

B. Pigmentation and Deposits

Epithelial, linear iron deposits are an age-related finding known as the **Hudson-Stähli line** when horizontal in the lower third of the cornea, or in keratoconus running circularly around the base of the cone (**Fleischer ring**), as a brown, vertical line in front of a pterygium (**Stocker line**) or directly in front of a filtering bleb (**Ferry line**). A circular, peripherally located golden-brown corneal ring at the level of Descemet's membrane (**Kayser-Fleischer ring, Ba**) is pathognomonic of copper deposition in Wilson disease. Corneal opacities due to dermatan, keratan, heparan, and keratan sulfate are found to varying degrees in young patients affected with the mucopolysaccharidoses. Treatment with chloroquine and amiodarone, as in Fabry disease, can lead to whorl-shaped deposits (**cornea verticillata**). **Corneal crystals** develop because of gold therapy (chrysiasis), in cystinosis (**Bb**), and in monoclonal gammopathies.

C. Thygeson Keratitis and Recurrent Corneal Erosions

Thygeson keratitis (**C**) shows bilateral, superficial, snowflake-like, stainable epithelial opacities of unknown cause. Treatment is prolonged with local steroids, tear substitutes, or cyclosporin A eye drops. The disease resolves spontaneously. **Recurrent corneal erosions** may occur from local corneal disease or after superficial corneal trauma. Clinically there is sudden unilateral pain, blepharospasm, photophobia, and epiphora. Slit-lamp examination shows a noninflamed corneal epithelial defect.

Tear substitutes and contact lenses are used therapeutically, and possibly also phototherapeutic keratectomy, corneal needling, or epithelial débridement.

D. Neurogenic Degeneration

Diseases of the trigeminal nerve lead to anesthesia of the corneal epithelium with the development of neuroparalytic keratitis. Clinically, punctate keratitis occurs first, with slow development of corneal edema. **Lagophthalmic keratitis** (**D**) is exposure keratitis due to incomplete lid closure in facial palsy.

E. Corneal Dystrophies

The corneal dystrophies are bilateral, symmetrical, progressive disorders of cell function and morphology. They are usually due to dominant inheritance and commence in youth. They are classified according to the preferred corneal layer into epithelial, Bowman's membrane, stromal, and endothelial dystrophies, or according to the gene locus, which is usually known today. Glare and reduced vision are the clinically predominant symptoms. Recurrent painful erosions occur in the epithelial dystrophies. These dystrophies are treated with tear substitutes and therapeutic contact lenses. With increasing loss of vision, lamellar or penetrating keratoplasty is indicated in all of the dystrophies.

A. Degeneration in Systemic Diseases

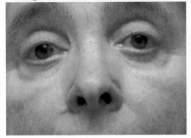

a Skin appearance in rosacea

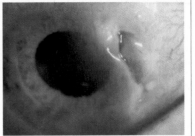

b Keratitis in rheumatoid arthritis

B. Pigmentation and Deposits

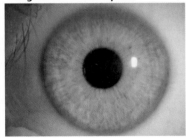

a Kayser-Fleischer ring

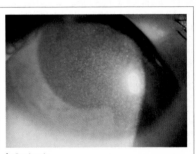

b Cystinosis

C. Thygeson Keratitis and Recurrent Corneal Erosions

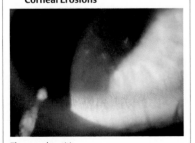

Thygeson keratitis

D. Neurogenic Degeneration

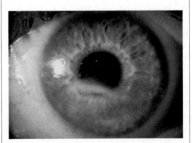

Lagophthalmic keratitis

Degenerative Conditions, Dystrophies

A. Meesmann Dystrophy

Etiology/pathogenesis. Mutations of the keratin genes 3 and 12 on chromosomes 12q13 and 17q12 lead to tiny 10–50 μm keratin-filled microcysts.

Clinical features. Bilateral, multiple, whitish, transparent, very delicate epithelial vesicles sharply demarcated from the uninvolved epithelium. Vision is preserved for a long time. Erosions.

Differential diagnosis. Microcystic dystrophy, band-shaped or whorl-shaped dystrophy. Prognosis. Slow course. Rapid recurrence after surgical treatment.

B. Microcystic Epithelial Dystrophy (Cogan, Map-Dot-Fingerprint Dystrophy)

Etiology/pathogenesis. Thickening of the basement membrane. PAS-positive cysts migrate from the basement membrane to the surface.

Epidemiology. Women > men.

Clinical features. Four different forms of epithelial opacity are described (maps, dots, fingerprints, vesicles). The clinical appearance is variable. The condition is usually asymptomatic. Astigmatism, corneal erosions, blurred vision, and foreign-body sensation occur (**Ba, b**).

Differential diagnosis. Meesmann dystrophy, band-shaped or whorl-shaped dystrophy.

Treatment. Phototherapeutic keratectomy.

Prognosis. Recurrences.

C. Honeycomb Dystrophy (Thiel-Behnke)

Etiology/pathogenesis. Mutation of the keratoepithelin gene on chromosome 5q31 or on chromosome 10q23–24. Dystrophy of Bowman's membrane.

Clinical features. In the early stage, diffuse subepithelial opacity; later honeycomb or fishnet pattern. Opacity-free zone ca. 1 mm toward the limbus. Recurrent painful erosions in childhood. Reduction in vision in adulthood.

Differential diagnosis. Reis-Bücklers dystrophy.

Prognosis. Recurrences in the graft within five years.

D. Reis-Bücklers Dystrophy (Granular Corneal Dystrophy Type III)

Etiology/pathogenesis. Mutation of the keratoepithelin gene on chromosome 5q31, which leads to subepithelial hyaline deposits and destruction of Bowman's membrane.

Epidemiology. Very rare. Full manifestation of the disease in the second decade of life.

Clinical features. Dense, gray-white, sharply demarcated subepithelial, maplike opacities with lighter and denser areas. "Lunar landscape." Periphery free. Painful erosions in childhood, which persist with aging. Severe reduction in vision.

Differential diagnosis. Honeycomb dystrophy. Prognosis. Recurrences in the graft within five years, usually above Bowman's membrane.

E. Granular Dystrophy Type I (Groenouw I)

Epidemiology. Most frequent form of granular dystrophy.

Clinical features. Small (<300 μm), gray-white, sharply demarcated granules in a fan shape under the epithelium in otherwise clear stroma. The limbus remains free. Photophobia, erosions in 50 % of adults, reduction in vision. Can have a long asymptomatic course (**Ea, b**).

Differential diagnosis. Reis-Bücklers dystrophy. **Prognosis.** Recurrences in the graft after 1–2 years. They are then situated between the epithelium and Bowman's membrane.

F. Lattice Dystrophy Type I

Etiology/pathogenesis. There are five known different mutations of the keratoepithelin gene on chromosome 5q31. Pathological keratoepithelin is deposited subepithelially and in the anterior stroma.

Epidemiology. Manifestation in the first decade.

Clinical features. Irregular, fine, semitransparent, radial lines forming lattice patterns. Point and diffuse opacities beside them. The patient complains of recurrent erosions. Development of astigmatism and reduction in vision are possible. Variable severity.

Prognosis. Recurrences in the graft always occur.

A. Meesmann Dystrophy

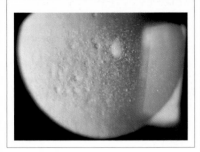

B. Microcystic Epithelial Dystrophy

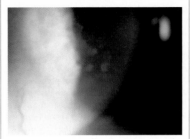

a Cogan dot dystrophy

E. Granular Dystrophy Type I

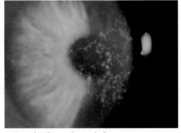

a Granular dystrophy, early form

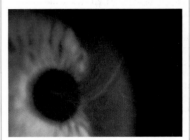

b Cogan fingerprint dystrophy

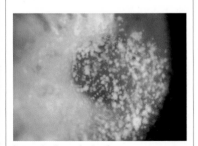

b Granular dystrophy, late form

F. Lattice Dystrophy Type I

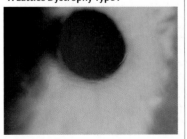

Lattice dystrophy

A. Macular Dystrophy

Etiology/pathogenesis. A mutation on chromosome 16q22 is suspected. Autosomal-recessive inheritance. Disorder of keratan sulfate synthesis.

Clinical features. Bilateral, blotchy corneal opacities involving several corneal layers and the limbus. Diffuse opacities and pseudoguttae. In the full condition there is complete opacity of the stroma. Signs occur between the ages of 5 and 10 years. Reduction in vision even at a young age.

Prognosis. Recurrences in the graft only after years.

B. Central Crystalline Dystrophy of Schnyder

Etiology/pathogenesis. Unclear. Gene locus 1p34.1–p36. Inflammation-free deposition of cholesterol and phospholipids in the basement membrane, Bowman's membrane, and stroma.

Epidemiology. Very rare.

Clinical features. Bilateral, crystalline, polychromatic corneal deposits in the anterior stroma, subsequently central discoid opacities. Arcus senilis. Association with disorders of lipid metabolism not certain.

Differential diagnosis. Lecithin cholesterol acetyltransferase deficiency, fish-eye disease, Tangier disease.

Treatment. Penetrating keratoplasty necessary very rarely.

Prognosis. Good overall.

C. Cornea Guttata/Fuchs Endothelial Dystrophy

Etiology/pathogenesis. Autosomal dominant disease of the pump function of the endothelial cells is assumed; reduced endothelial cell density.

Epidemiology. Women are affected four times more often than men. The disease commences after the age of 40 years.

Clinical features. Wartlike thickenings of Descemet's membrane. In regressive light the back of the cornea can have a "beaten metal" appearance. Depending on the stage, reduction in vision, photophobia, and pain when vesicles burst. Often improvement in symptoms in the course of the day because of physiological evaporation.

Course in 4 stages:
1. Cornea guttata
2. Epithelial and stromal edema (C)
3. Bullous keratopathy
4. Vascularization, scarring, superinfection

Differential diagnosis. In stage 1, Hassall-Henle corpuscles.

D. Congenital Hereditary Endothelial Dystrophy (CHED)

Etiology/pathogenesis. Mutation in the pericentric region of chromosome 20p11.2–q11.2.

Clinical features. Occurs in childhood. Bilateral whitish corneal opacity, no vascularization or signs of inflammation. Band degeneration and development of pannus. Thin, defective Descemet's membrane with absence of endothelial cells, corneal edema, and loss of vision. The dominant form (CHED I) shows a clear cornea at birth; the recessive form (CHED II) shows early corneal opacities.

Differential diagnosis. Posterior polymorphic dystrophy of Schlichting.

E. Posterior Polymorphic Dystrophy (Schlichting Corneal Dystrophy)

Etiology/pathogenesis. Mutation in the pericentromeric region of chromosome 20. It is suspected that this is a different phenotype of congenital hereditary endothelial dystrophy.

Clinical features. Circumscribed, bilateral alterations that are subdivided into three forms biomicroscopically: vesicular, geographic, and curvilinear opacities in the endothelium. Descemet's membrane is thickened and may be opacified and gray. Usually asymptomatic coincidental finding. Corneal decompensation with severe endothelial involvement; there is then also a frequent association with glaucoma or anterior chamber angle anomalies.

Differential diagnosis. Congenital hereditary endothelial dystrophy.

Treatment. Almost never requires treatment.

Prognosis. Good. The disease can recur in a graft. Spontaneous remission is possible.

A. Macular Dystrophy

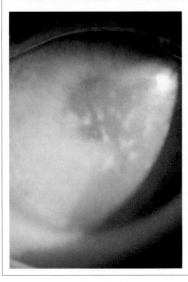

B. Central Crystalline Dystrophy of Schnyder

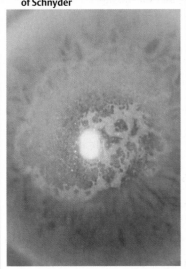

C. Cornea Guttata/Fuchs Endothelial Dystrophy

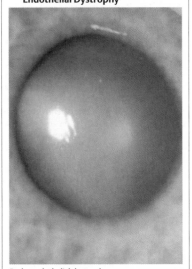

Fuchs endothelial dystrophy

E. Posterior Polymorphic Dystrophy (Schlichting Corneal Dystrophy)

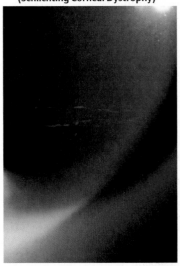

A. Keratoconus

Etiology/pathogenesis. Dystrophy with development of a defect of the collagen in Bowman's membrane and central corneal thinning.

Epidemiology. The disease has an increased familial incidence and can be associated with neurodermatitis, Down syndrome, Turner syndrome, Marfan syndrome, and Ehlers-Danlos syndrome.

Clinical features. The corneal surface has an asymmetrical, pointed-spherical shape, bilateral (**Aa**) with vertical lines in the stroma (Vogt lines). Tears of Descemet's membrane can lead to sudden corneal decompensation ("acute keratoconus," **Ab**). Reduction in vision and changes in refraction occur episodically with the development of myopic irregular astigmatism. Slit-lamp examination shows a hemosiderin ring (Fleischer ring) around the base of the keratoconus.

Diagnosis. The protrusion is seen from the side or from above (Munson's sign, **Ac**). Corneal topography is used to make the diagnosis and monitor progress (**Ad**). It is classified as slight (>48 D), moderate (>54 D), or severe (>54 D).

Differential diagnosis. Megalocornea, buphthalmos.

Treatment. Fitting of rigid contact lenses. If correction of the astigmatism is no longer possible, penetrating keratoplasty is indicated when there is increasing reduction in vision.

Prognosis. The disease progresses but then comes to a halt in two-thirds of cases. It is argued that the disease recurs after penetrating keratoplasty.

B. Other Ectatic Dystrophies

Keratoglobus (**B**) is a severe disease already present at birth. There is thinning of the entire cornea, which is greatest peripherally. There is a risk of rupture. The back of the cornea projects spherically. In the rare **pellucid marginal degeneration**, a paracentral inferior area of cornea becomes thinned. The cornea above it protrudes.

C. Infections of the Cornea

Infections due to viruses, bacteria, fungi, and protozoa are the most frequent form of keratitis. In contrast, mechanical, toxic, radiological, degenerative, dystrophic, and neurotrophic keratitides are rarer. Scars develop in ulcerating keratitis when Bowman's membrane is destroyed. Purely epithelial keratitis heals without scarring. In nonulcerating processes and when the epithelium is intact, scars arise through neovascularization, resolution of collagen fibers, or endothelial decompensation.

D. Bacterial Keratitis

Etiology/pathogenesis. *Staphylococcus aureus, Staphylococcus epidermidis, Streptococcus pneumoniae, Pseudomonas aeruginosa, Moraxella.*

Epidemiology. Wearers of contact lenses or patients with diseases of the corneal surface (previous trauma, sicca syndrome, lid deformities, etc.) are particularly at risk.

Clinical features. Pain, photophobia, epiphora, blepharospasm, mucopurulent secretion, corneal ulcer (**D**), corneal infiltrate, reduction in vision, hypopyon. Although the clinical signs are not typical of the pathogen, staphylococcal and streptococcal infections often show dense, oval, yellow-white opacities. *Pseudomonas* infections lead to sharply demarcated, rapidly progressive ulcers.

Diagnosis. Clinical appearance, conjunctival swab with antibiotic sensitivity, scrapings. Differential diagnosis. Keratitis from other causes.

Treatment. Treatment according to antibiotic sensitivity. Not longer than 10 days, as otherwise no epithelial closure will occur. In severe cases, it is necessary to make up highly concentrated antibiotics for topical/subconjunctival use. "Hot" keratoplasty if perforationis threatened. If there is concomitant iritis, a mydriatic should be used.

Prognosis. Perforation is possible within 48 h with *Pseudomonas aeruginosa*. Depending on the size and position of the defect, a reduction in vision, scarring, and astigmatism are possible.

A. Keratoconus

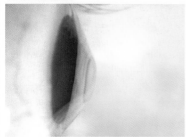

a Keratoconus

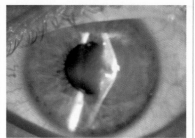

b Acute keratoconus

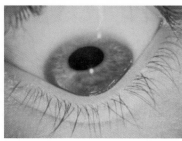

c Munson's sign

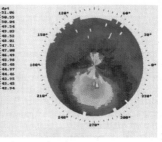

d Corneal topography in keratoconus

B. Other Ectatic Dystrophies

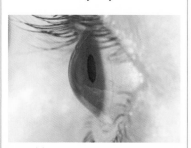

Keratoglobus

D. Bacterial Keratitis

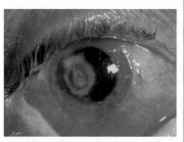

Bacterial corneal ulcer

A. Herpes Simplex Keratitis

Etiology/pathogenesis. Herpes simplex virus (HSV) type 1. Local recurrences occur, e. g., with general infections, pyrexia, sun exposure, immunosuppression, and menstruation.

Epidemiology. Very common infection. The primary infection occurs from the age of 6 months. Infection is present in about 90 % of the population.

Clinical features. The primary infection in the eye is similar to unilateral follicular conjunctivitis with swelling of the preauricular lymph nodes. Rapidly crusting vesicles are found on the lids and periorbital skin.

Keratitis is fundamentally a recurrence. HSV infection can have the appearance of epithelial, endothelial or stromal keratitis. The typical appearance is of dendritic or geographic keratitis (**Aa**). Corneal sensitivity is reduced. Rarely, the disease leads to necrotic stromal infiltration with folds in Descemet's membrane, edema, and inflammation of the anterior segment of the eye with secondary glaucoma (**Ab**). Retinitis occurs predominantly in immunosuppressed patients (see Chapter 13). Disciform keratitis (metaherpetic keratitis, endotheliitis, Ac) is a collective term for immune complex reactions that are not viral in origin (corneal edema, folds in Descemet's membrane, infiltrations).

Diagnosis. Clinical appearance, esthesiometry, fluorescein staining, measurement of ocular pressure.

Differential diagnosis. Red eye, keratitis from other causes.

Treatment. Aciclovir eye ointment 5 times a day, atropine 1 % twice a day, continued until three days after healing. Partial scraping when there is purely epithelial involvement. In disciform keratitis, local treatment; with simultaneous kerato-uveitis or inflammatory secondary glaucoma, aciclovir 800 mg 5 times a day for three weeks. Systemic therapy for a period of up to 12 months is recommended. Steroids should be given only after epithelial closure and only for a short time; they reduce scarring in stromal keratitis. Penetrating keratoplasty should be performed with aciclovir cover only if there has previously been freedom from recurrence for 6–12 months.

Prognosis. The primary infection is often self-limiting. Recurrences also heal spontaneously after 2–3 weeks. Antiviral therapy shortens the duration of the disease.

B. Herpes Zoster Keratitis

Etiology/pathogenesis. The cause of the disease is human herpes virus type 3, which causes both chickenpox and zoster. Due to the viremia in chickenpox, a few virus particles persist in the nerve ganglia. Endogenous reinfection originating in the gasserian ganglion occurs in the territory of the trigeminal nerve.

Epidemiology. The disease can occur at any age, but elderly persons and immunosuppressed patients are mostly affected. Shingles occurs in about 20 % of the population, with eye involvement in 15–20 %.

Clinical features. Sudden, very painful onset of the disease, usually before the visible exanthem. All the divisions of the trigeminal nerve can be affected. The conjunctiva is often also involved. However, involvement of the lids, cornea, sclera, uveal tract, and retina is possible. Corneal disease is manifested primarily as punctate keratitis or as dendritic ulcers. Corneal reactions can occur such as those of herpes simplex keratitis. Anterior stromal infiltrates also appear in one-third of cases about 10 days after the start of the disease. Disciform keratitis occurs three weeks after the onset of the disease. Corneal sensation is abolished.

Diagnosis. Clinical appearance, tonometry, examination of motility.

Differential diagnosis. Herpes simplex keratitis, conjunctivitis.

Treatment. Oral aciclovir; alternatively, valaciclovir or famciclovir.

Prognosis. If scarring occurs, lid deformities are possible. A few patients suffer from severe chronic pain. Not infrequently, lipid keratopathy develops later.

A. Herpes Simplex Keratitis

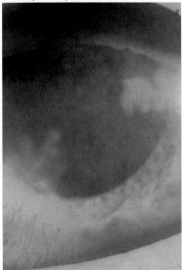

a Dendritic keratitis and geographic keratitis

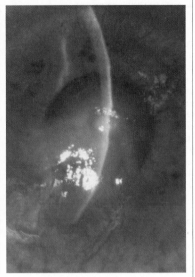

b Corneal ulcer in herpes simplex

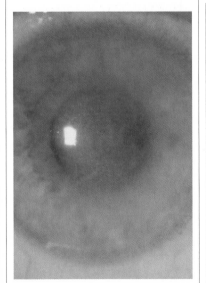

c Metaherpetic keratitis

B. Herpes Zoster Keratitis

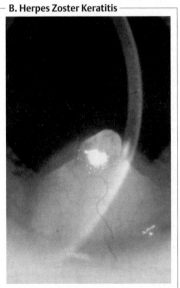

Lipid keratopathy in herpes zoster

A. Epidemic Keratitis

Etiology/pathogenesis. Infection with highly infectious adenoviruses type 8 and 19. Route of transmission: hand-eye.

Epidemiology. No age or sex predisposition.

Clinical features. Rapid unilateral onset with epiphora, follicular conjunctivitis, swelling of plica and caruncle, chemosis, blepharospasm, sticky eyes, lymph node swelling. Within a short time the second eye is affected also. Typically, the following course is seen in the cornea:

- Diffuse epithelial keratitis
- Punctate keratitis
- Stromal opacities
- Subepithelial infiltrates (**A**) with reduction in vision and photophobia

Diagnosis. Clinical appearance. Rapid testing.

Differential diagnosis. Herpes simplex keratoconjunctivitis, Thygeson superficial keratitis, chlamydial infection, molluscum contagiosum. Treatment. Further spread must be avoided by handwashing and disinfection. Artificial tears. Antibiotic eye drops only in superinfection.

Prognosis. The incubation period is 8–9 days. Patients are still infectious 14 days after the onset of the disease. The conjunctivitis lasts for about two weeks. It takes months before the disease is cured and persistence of the corneal infiltrates for years is possible.

B. Acanthamoeba Keratitis

Etiology/pathogenesis. Acanthamoebas are ubiquitous protozoa. They are present in the form of a replicating trophozoite that is motile and as a resting cyst. The cystic form in particular is very resistant and can survive in swimming pools, hot water, and also in ice. Epidemiology. Wearers of soft contact lenses or patients after corneal trauma are frequently affected.

Clinical features. Glare, reduction in vision, severe pain. Recurrent, fluorescein-positive epithelial defects, multilocular stromal infiltrates (ring infiltrates). The infiltrates have a dendritic appearance but are subepithelial in location. Diffuse anterior scleritis or uveitis.

Diagnosis. Smear. Scrapings. Culture on agar enriched with E. coli. Double-walled polygonal cysts on H/E or PAS staining. Examine contact lenses at the same time.

Differential diagnosis. The disease is easily confused with herpes simplex keratitis or with fungal keratitis.

Treatment. Intensive local antibiotics or biguanides.

Prognosis. Protracted course with remissions and recurrences.

C. Fungal Keratitis

Etiology/pathogenesis. Fungal keratitides occurs after ocular trauma due to the introduction of plant materials into the eye. These are usually *Aspergillus fusarium* and *Cephalosporium species*. In debilitated or immunosuppressed patients fungal infections tend rather to be caused by *Candida* and other yeasts.

Epidemiology. These are rare diseases.

Clinical features. The clinical appearance resembles bacterial keratitis. There is a gray-white infiltrate with fine "outliers" in the stroma (**satellite lesions, Ca, b**). Hypopyon is often found. The condition worsens when steroids are given.

Diagnosis. The history is instructive. If there is no response to antibiotic therapy, fungal keratitis should be considered. Corneal sensitivity is reduced. Scrapings from the margin of the ulcer can be examined histologically.

Differential diagnosis. Bacterial keratitis.

Treatment. Local administration of natamycin eye ointment. Change to alternative preparations if necessary. Mydriatics if there is anterior chamber irritation. Systemic treatment with ketoconazole is occasionally indicated.

Prognosis. Usually a slow healing process. In some cases a penetrating keratoplasty must be performed.

A. Epidemic Keratitis

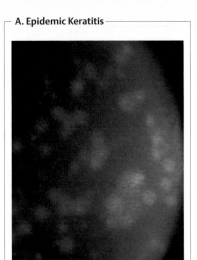

Subepithelial infiltrates

B. Acanthamoeba Keratitis

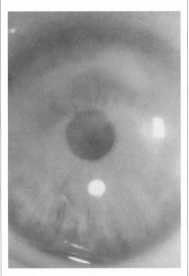

C. Fungal Keratitis

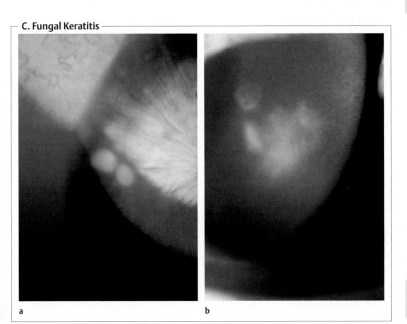

a

b

A. Corneal Trauma

A distinction can be made according to the source of injury into mechanical, electromagnetic (UV) radiation, thermal, or chemical trauma. The most common forms of trauma are corneal foreign bodies and traumatic corneal erosions/abrasions. The treatment and prognosis depend on the extent of the trauma. Penetrating and perforating injuries require thorough investigation and mainly surgical management.

B. UV keratopathy

This is injury due to UV radiation, e.g., during welding or high-altitude exposure. After a latency of 6–8 hours, patients develop a reduction in vision with pain, blepharospasm, epiphora, and a foreign-body sensation. Clinically, unilateral or bilateral **superficial punctate keratitis** (**B**) is seen in the region of the palpebral fissure. Depending on the history, a corneal foreign body must be considered in the differential diagnosis. Tear substitutes and gentamicin eye drops t.i.d. are helpful in treatment. Despite the dramatic clinical picture ("sunburn of the eye"), it is a harmless superficial injury that heals without sequelae.

C. Chemical Injury/Burns

Etiology/pathogenesis. Injury due to alkali, acid, or heat (**Ca, b**). The severity of the injury depends on the agent, its concentration, and the duration of exposure. Alkali burns cause greater damage than acid burns. The coagulation necrosis caused by an acid burn prevents further penetration of the acid. The colliquation necrosis of an alkali burn leads to rapid penetration of the alkali into the anterior segment of the eye.

Epidemiology. Frequent occupational injury; 7–10% of all eye injuries. A large proportion of the patients are young working men between 20 and 40 years of age. The ratio of acid to alkali burn is about 1 : 2 to 1 : 3.

Clinical features. The acute phase is associated initially with a varying degree of loss of vision, pain, epiphora, and blepharospasm.

Clinically, the extent of the burn can be divided into four stages (after Reim):

I   Corneal erosion, clear cornea, hyperemia, intact perilimbal vessels

II   Corneal erosion, slight clouding of the cornea, ischemia of the limbus region > ⅓ of the circumference, chemosis (**Cc**).

III   Corneal erosion, clouding of the cornea, ischemia of the limbus region > ½ of the circumference, ulceration, development of pannus, stromal neovascularization, scarring (**Cd**).

IV   Corneal erosion, ischemia of the limbus region > ¾ of the circumference, necrosis, ulcers, symblephara, scarring, lid deformities, secondary glaucoma, cataract, hypotension, phthisis bulbi.

Diagnosis. Diagnosis is made from the history. The staging is guided by the clinical picture. Intraocular structures in the anterior segment of the eye can also be involved and can be associated with lens opacities and secondary glaucoma.

Treatment. Immediate irrigation of the eye is the most important first aid measure.

Prognosis. The prognosis of the disease depends critically on how rapidly irrigation is performed. Regeneration of the corneal epithelium depends on the extent of the damage to limbal stem cells. Epithelialization by the stem cells does not take place if more than half of the circumference of the limbus is damaged. Rather, conjunctival tissue grows over the defect.

D. Superglue (Cyanoacrylate) Injuries

If rapid-setting adhesive gets into the eye, it hardens on the cornea and falls off (**D**). The resulting corneal erosion is treated with tear substitutes and local antibiotics. The condition usually heals without sequelae.

B. UV keratopathy

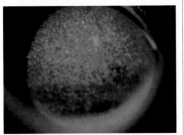

Superficial punctate keratitis (stained with fluorescein)

D. Superglue Injury

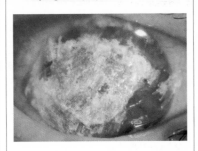

C. Chemical Injury/Burns

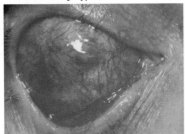

a Following burn from hot aluminum: conjunctivalization of the corneal surface

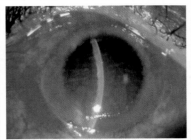

b Acid burn with corneal erosion below

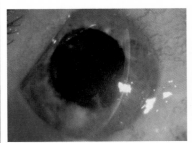

c Alkali burn stage II

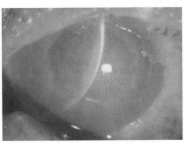

d Alkali burn stage III

A. Superficial/Penetrating/Perforating Injuries

Etiology/pathogenesis. The pattern of injury varies and ranges from erosion, a superficial loss of epithelium, through lamellar injuries and foreign-body penetration (**Aa–c**) to perforating injuries with involvement of the inner structures of the eye or even loss of the eye.

Epidemiology. The injuries occur in association with occupational or leisure activities. Men aged between 20 and 40 years are predominantly affected. Corneal foreign bodies are the most frequent ocular injuries and the greatest proportion of corneal foreign bodies consists of metal. Only about 5 % are of an organic nature.

Clinical features. Usually pain, epiphora, blepharospasm, conjunctivitis, upper lid swelling, and reduction in vision. However, the symptoms can also sometimes be very slight and visual acuity is preserved fully. If there is hyphema and a rise in intraocular pressure, the stromal part of the cornea becomes stained after 48 hours. The cause of hematocornea (**Ad**) is hemoglobin and other breakdown products of the erythrocytes.

Diagnosis. Diagnosis is made from the history and thorough examination with lid eversion, staining of the cornea, inspection of the wound with the operating microscope, and if necessary radiography of the orbit in two planes or CT.

Treatment. Operative removal of the foreign body and wound closure. Local or systemic antibiotics. If necessary, second operation for injuries of intraocular structures.

Prognosis. Depends on type of injury.

B. Corneal Changes after Surgery

Corneal changes following phacoemulsification include folds in Descemet's membrane, lysis of Descemet's membrane, and "snail tracks." Injuries of the endothelium can lead to endothelial decompensation with development of bullous keratopathy. Penetrating keratoplasty is then indicated.

Silicone oil keratopathy occurs in vitreoretinal surgery when there is prolonged contact between silicone oil and corneal endothelium. The keratopathy develops within months and is usually associated with secondary glaucoma. Clinically the appearance is of increasingly dense whitish stromal opacification of the cornea.

C. Corneal Changes after Refractive Surgery

Corneal operations to correct refractive errors lead to typical corneal changes depending on the procedure. In radial keratotomy (**Ca**), 80–90 % of the thickness of the cornea is incised radially. This procedure was introduced to correct myopia but has now been replaced by laser refractive correction methods. **Photorefractive keratectomy** (**PRK**) removes superficial layers of the cornea with the excimer laser and produces correction of myopia when the central cornea is flattened or correction of hyperopia when the curvature of the cornea is increased. A possible side-effect is the development of a central corneal scar (**haze, Cb**). In **laser in situ keratomileusis** (**LASIK**) a layer of ca. 130 µm of cornea (**flap**) is raised. The underlying cornea is flattened with the excimer laser and the flap is replaced. Loss of the flap, clouding or dislocation of the flap, ingrowth of epithelium, or infectious keratitis are rare adverse effects of the procedure. Laser epithelial keratomileusis (**LASEK**) combines the techniques of both of these procedures. A so-called epithelial flap is raised and an excimer laser ablation is performed underneath this. The epithelium is then replaced. All of the procedures lead to falsely low measurements of the intraocular pressure and effect the calculation of an artificial lens.

A. Superficial/Penetrating/Perforating Injuries

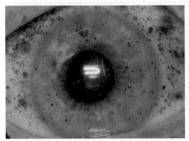

a Explosive injury

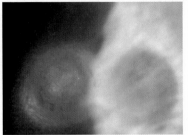

b Corneal siderosis due to iron-containing foreign body

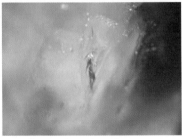

c Lamellar injury due to glass splinter

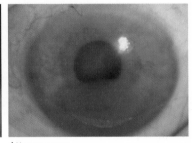

d Hematocornea

C. Corneal Changes after Refractive Surgery

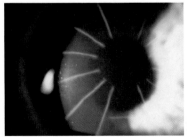

a Radial keratotomy

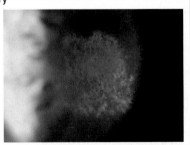

b Haze after photorefractive keratectomy

A. Keratoplasty

In **penetrating keratoplasty** all the layers of the cornea are transplanted from a donor to a recipient, whereas in **lamellar keratoplasty** the deep stroma, Descemet's membrane, and the endothelium are left in the recipient.

The most frequent indications for penetrating keratoplasty are bullous keratopathy, keratoconus, corneal dystrophy, corneal scarring that has occurred after infectious keratitis or trauma, and re-keratoplasties. The circular graft is fitted into a correspondingly sized trepanned recipient bed, typically with two continuous cross sutures (**Aa**).

In **tectonic keratoplasty** (**Ab**), restoration of visual function is not the principal aim but rather preservation of the globe. Alternatively, threatened perforation can be covered by amniotic membrane. **Keratoplasty à chaud** means keratoplasty performed as an emergency. As the cornea is a bradytrophic, avascular tissue, there is a particular immunological situation. Prior to transplantation, it is not necessary to ensure strict tissue compatibility as in the case of other organs. Nevertheless, HLA typing should be performed in high-risk keratoplasties. In order to avoid the risk of graft failure, keratoplasty must be strictly indicated. Lid deformities, dry eye, glaucoma, and poor compliance are contraindications.

B. Complications of Keratoplasty

Immunological transplant reactions can occur even years after the operation. The rejection reactions are classified according to their location in the corneal tissue. The **epithelial rejection reaction** consists of a slightly raised stainable line of cytotoxic lymphocytes running centrally from the edge of the graft (**epithelial Khodadoust line**). This form of immune reaction is usually not dangerous. **Subepithelial changes** often occur months after the transplantation. These appear as irregular subepithelial infiltrates on the graft and appear similar to the infiltrates in adenoviral keratoconjunctivitis. The eye is otherwise completely uninflamed. They are often a coincidental finding, which is reversible provided deeper layers of the cornea are not involved. With stromal changes, superficial graft coalescence can occur, and acute **stromal necrosis** occurs in 1–2 %. This is a dense whitish infiltration by leukocytes, lympho-

cytes, and plasma cells affecting all the layers of the cornea. An infectious corneal ulcer must be considered in the differential diagnosis. **Endothelial changes** have a heterogeneous appearance clinically. As in the epithelium, a line running from the edge of the graft to the center of cytotoxic lymphocytes can be seen in the focally progressive endothelial reaction. This so-called **endothelial Khodadoust** line moves at a varying rate and separates the endothelium that has been destroyed by lymphocytes from the still intact graft (**Ba**). In the diffuse immune reaction, disseminated precipitates are found on the endothelium. The endothelial immune reactions lead to corneal edema. In addition, **nonimmunological causes** can lead to graft failure (**Bb**). These include poor wound apposition and delayed wound healing at the edge of the graft, dry eye, infections (**Bc**), toxic medication damage, ingrowth of epithelial vessels, and recurrences of the underlying disease. The last has been described with herpes simplex keratitis (**Bd**), keratoconus, and the corneal dystrophies. Surgical procedures can also trigger a rejection reaction. The treatment is guided by the cause of the graft damage and includes tear substitutes, contact lenses, antibiotics, antiviral drugs or immunosuppressants, or re-keratoplasty. Before instituting therapy, the epithelial toxicity of the individual substances should be considered.

A. Keratoplasty

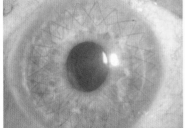

a Continuous running suture in keratoplasty

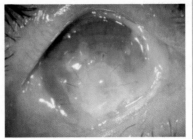

b Opacified tectonic keratoplasty

B. Complications of Keratoplasty

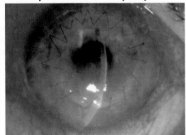

a Endothelial Khodadoust line

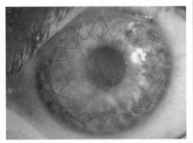

b Graft failure

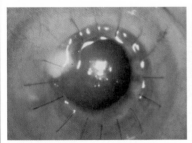

c Suture infection

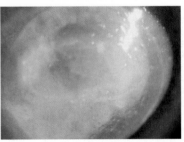

d Herpes simplex recurrence on graft

A. Malformations and Anomalies

A blue sclera can occur in isolation as an inherited autosomal dominant or recessive anomaly. It is seen in keratoconus and keratoglobus in association with other ocular diseases and is also a partial aspect of various hereditary systemic diseases such as osteogenesis imperfecta (types 1–4), Ehlers-Danlos syndrome, Marfan syndrome, and Turner syndrome. The normal fetal transparency of the sclera is preserved.

Alkaptonuria (ochronosis) is due to an inherited autosomal recessive deficiency of the enzyme homogentisate oxidase and leads to deposition of homogentisic acid especially in cartilage and other avascular connective tissue. Spotty black deposits are seen in the conjunctiva, cornea, and sclera in about 70 % of patients.

Sclerectasia and **scleral staphylomas** can occur as isolated congenital malformations. Whereas sclerectasia is purely a bulging out of the sclera, scleral staphylomas are local areas of thinning that reveal underlying uveal tissue.

B. Degenerative Conditions and Age-related Changes

Age-related scleral atrophy with bluish uveal tissue showing through can be observed in many people at an advanced age and is of no pathological significance. This includes **senile hyaline scleral plaques (Ba)**, which become visible as oval alterations in front of the attachments of the horizontal extraocular muscles and are the result of local calcification. Treatment is not necessary.

The causes of acquired sclerectasia or staphyloma are congenital glaucoma/buphthalmos, injury, scleritis, uveitis, degenerative myopia, or surgical procedures. Excessively progressive degenerative myopia leads to sclerectasia circumscribed behind or **posterior staphyloma (Bb)**. This is a sharply demarcated bulging of the entire posterior pole, which is associated with massive chorioretinal atrophy.

C. Episcleritis

Episcleritis is an inflammation of the episclera, a loose, highly vascularized connective tissue immediately on the surface of the sclera. Diffuse (**Ca**) and nodular forms (**Cb**) are distinguished.

Etiology/pathogenesis. The majority of cases of episcleritis are idiopathic. A systemic disease, usually of an autoimmune nature, it is present in ca. 35 % (**C, Table 1**). Local infections or corrosive injuries are less common.

Epidemiology. Not uncommon. Young and middle-aged adults and especially women are mainly affected. Bilateral in 30–35 %.

Clinical features. The onset is usually acute, with red eye, epiphora, and mild to moderate pain. There is less tenderness than with scleritis. The appearance of diffuse episcleritis is of a variable, extensive, and edematous episclera with congestion of the superficial episcleral vascular plexus. Nodular episcleritis shows one or more circumscribed nodular thickenings of the episclera with increased vascular injection. The nodules are mobile on the sclera.

Diagnosis. The diagnosis is made clinically. A full medical and dermatological examination should be performed, especially when there is systemic disease or recurrence (**C, Table 1**). Infections (syphilis) and metabolic disorders (gout) should be excluded.

Differential diagnosis. Conjunctivitis, scleritis.

Treatment. Treat any associated systemic disease. Mild, idiopathic episcleritis without symptoms can be observed. More severe disease can be treated with short-term local corticosteroids and systemic nonsteroidal anti-inflammatory drugs. High-dose oral corticosteroid therapy is necessary only rarely.

Prognosis. Usually mild, self-limiting course (1–2 weeks). Frequency of recurrence ca. 30 %. Ocular complications are rarer than with scleritis: anterior uveitis (12 %), corneal involvement (15 %), secondary glaucoma (4–8 %).

B. Degenerative Conditions and Age-related Changes

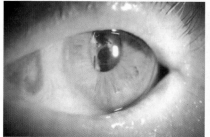

a Senile scleral plaques

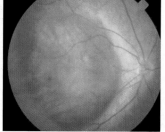

b Posterior staphyloma

C. Episcleritis

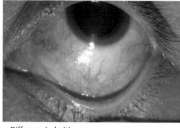

a Diffuse episcleritis

b Nodular episcleritis

Table 1 Systemic diseases with episcleritis

Joints	Rheumatoid arthritis Seronegative spondyloarthropathies
Connective tissue	Systemic lupus erythematosus Recurrent polychondritis
Vasculitis	Behçet disease Polyarteritis nodosa Giant-cell arteritis Wegener granulomatosis Cogan syndrome II
Infectious/granulomatous	Syphilis Tuberculosis Herpes simplex Sarcoidosis
Intestine	Ulcerative colitis Crohn disease
Skin	Rosacea Atopic dermatitis Ophthalmic zoster
Metabolic	Gout

A. Scleritis

Scleritis is a severe inflammation of the wall of the globe (sclera). A distinction is made between anterior scleritis (involvement of the anterior part of the sclera) and posterior scleritis. Anterior scleritis is classified as diffuse (**Aa**), nodular (**Ab**), necrotizing scleritis with inflammation (**Ac**), and necrotizing scleritis without inflammation (scleromalacia perforans, **Ad**).

Etiology/pathogenesis. Infectious scleritis (bacteria, viruses, fungi), necrotizing scleritis after ocular surgery, scleritis associated with vasculitis/systemic diseases, and idiopathic scleritis can be distinguished (**A, Table 1**). The last two are primary immune-mediated vasculitides.

Epidemiology. Scleritis is rare; women are affected slightly more often than men. It can occur at any age but there is an increased incidence between 40 and 60 years. Anterior scleritis is much more common (95 %) than posterior scleritis (5 %). Anterior scleritis is bilateral in 30–50 %, but in scleromalacia perforans bilateral involvement is seen in up to 80 %. One form of scleritis does not usually transform into a different form once it has become manifest. In about 57 % of all patients with scleritis an underlying systemic disease can be found; this is a collagenosis or vasculitis in 48 %. The most common associated systemic disease is rheumatoid arthritis.

Clinical features. Usually acute onset with severe lancinating eye pain, pain on movement, photophobia, epiphora, and redness of the eye. In diffuse anterior scleritis, a sectorally limited livid discoloration of the sclera with increased filling of deep and superficial episcleral and conjunctival vessels can be seen. The inflamed area is very tender. In anterior nodular scleritis there is circumscribed granulomatous thickening of the sclera with a surrounding concomitant inflammatory reaction. Anterior necrotizing scleritis with inflammation leads to progressive destruction of scleral tissue, accompanied by obvious inflammatory changes such as those that are also found in diffuse anterior scleritis. In contrast, scleromalacia perforans has the appearance of necrotizing scleritis, in which inflammatory phenomena such as redness and swelling of surrounding tissue or pain are hardly observed. The thinning of the sclera can progress to obvious sclerectasia.

Scleral perforation is rare. The clinical signs of posterior scleritis, along with the pain in the eye, are loss of vision, papilledema, retinal and choroid folds (**Ae**), **serous retinal detachment**, subretinal granuloma and choroid detachment. Diffuse anterior scleritis is often present at the same time.

Diagnosis. The diagnosis is made clinically. The thickening of the posterior sclera especially in posterior scleritis can be imaged using ultrasound. **An underlying systemic disease/vasculitis** should be excluded in every scleritis of unclear origin. Sarcoidosis, borreliosis, tuberculosis, and syphilis should also be excluded.

Differential diagnosis. Conjunctivitis, episcleritis, myositis, orbital pseudotumor. Rarely masquerade syndrome with malignant melanoma of the choroid, lymphoma, and multiple myeloma (posterior scleritis) or invasive squamous cell carcinoma of the conjunctiva (necrotizing anterior scleritis).

Treatment. This depends on the cause, the severity of the scleritis, and the presence of a systemic disease. Local therapy alone is not sufficient. Mild idiopathic scleritis can be treated initially with nonsteroidal anti-inflammatory drugs. If this is not enough, high-dose corticosteroids are given orally. If necessary, other immunosuppressants can be used (e.g., methotrexate). If there is a systemic disease, its treatment predominates.

Prognosis. Variable. Often chronic recurrent course. Accordingly, ocular complications are frequent, especially with necrotizing scleritis: loss of vision (40 %), anterior uveitis (40 %), peripheral ulcerative keratitis, glaucoma and cataract (each 15–20 %). Wegener granulomatosis in particular is associated with severe necrotizing scleritis.

A. Scleritis

Table 1 Underlying systemic diseases

Joints	– Rheumatoid arthritis – Polyarticular juvenile idiopathic arthritis (seropositive) – Seronegative spondyloarthropathies
Connective tissue	– Systemic lupus erythematosus – Recurrent polychondritis – IgA nephropathy
Vasculitis	– Behçet disease – Polyarteritis nodosa – Giant-cell arteritis – Wegener granulomatosis – Cogan syndrome II – Takayasu disease
Infectious/ granulo- matous	– Syphilis – Tuberculosis – Borreliosis – Sarcoidosis
Intestine	– Ulcerative colitis – Crohn disease
Skin	– Ophthalmic zoster – Porphyria – Pyoderma gangrenosum
Metabolic	– Gout

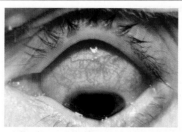

a Diffuse anterior scleritis

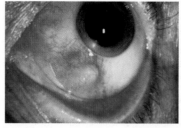

b Nodular anterior scleritis

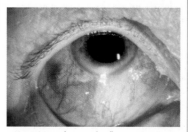

c Necrotizing scleritis with inflammation

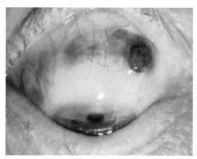

d Scleromalacia perforans

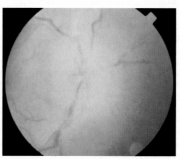

e Fundus appearance in posterior scleritis

A. Tumors

Primary tumors of the sclera are very rare. These include fibromas, fibrosarcomas, hemangiomas, epidermoids (**Aa**), neurofibromas, schwannomas, or ectopic lacrimal gland tissue. Benign episcleral osseous choristoma arises from ectopic bone tissue and is situated temporally above between the lateral and superior rectus muscles.

The sclera has only very slight pigmentation in caucasians (**Ab**). Pigment spots are seen especially with a dark iris and consist of episcleral collections of uveal melanocytes about 3–4 mm from the limbus, which have migrated from the uveal tract through scleral channels (ciliary arteries, intrascleral nerve loop of Axenfeld). They are of no pathological significance. Blue nevi of the sclera can occur in isolation. Conspicuous pigmentation of the sclera is seen together with increased pigmentation of other ocular structures (lids, uvea) in oculodermal melanocytosis (**Ota's nevus, Ac**) (see Chapter 10).

Secondary involvement of the sclera by ingrowth of malignant tumors of the conjunctiva (malignant melanoma, squamous cell carcinoma) or of the choroid (malignant melanoma) is more common than primary scleral tumors.

B. Surgical Changes and Trauma

Surgically induced necrotizing **sclerokeratitis** is a rare serious complication after ocular surgery. Patients who have had several ocular operations (cataract surgery, strabismus surgery, trabeculectomy, vitrectomy, buckle surgery) are affected in particular. It usually consists of necrotizing anterior scleritis, more rarely peripheral posterior scleritis, which is usually limited to the original area of operation. The scleritis manifests itself usually several months after the operation, more rarely after years. The etiology is unclear, but a hypersensitivity reaction to a scleral antigen released during operation and local ischemia have been suggested as initiating factors for an autoimmune reaction. In fact, a predisposing systemic disease (especially collagenosis) can be found in the majority of patients. Investigation must therefore be directed toward detecting a predisposing systemic disease (see p. 111, **Table 1**). The treatment should consist of oral administration of high-dose corticosteroids and other immunosuppressants if necessary. The tendency to recurrence is over 30%.

Besides the rather rare inflammatory conditions, many operations on the sclera lead to circumscribed **scleral atrophy** (**Ba**), which is usually without pathological significance but occasionally leads to sclerectasia. About 5% of all ocular traumas are associated with involvement of the sclera. This includes superficial and penetrating foreign bodies, sharp penetrating injury, and blunt trauma. Blunt trauma can lead to scleral rupture, where the tears occur mainly at the corneal limbus, the region of attachment of the external ocular muscles, or in the region of previous operative procedures. This applies particularly to cataract operated eyes, in which about 0.3% suffer traumatic wound dehiscence (**Bb**). With the corneoscleral approach to cataract operation, there is prolonged diminished postoperative wound strength: after one month it is about 30% of the initial strength and 75% after two years.

With every severe traumatic subconjunctival hemorrhage, an underlying scleral rupture must be considered (**Bc**). Indirect evidence consists of low ocular pressure, flattening or depression of the anterior chamber (compare sides), and the details of the accident. Foreign bodies and full-thickness defects can be imaged using ultrasound or CT. Scleral ruptures and tears require surgical management in order to restore stability to the globe, prevent infection inside the eye, and enable (later) internal reconstruction.

A. Tumors

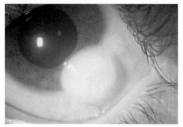

a Epidermoid

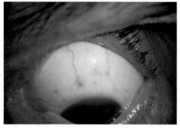

b Normal scleral pigmentation (pigment spots)

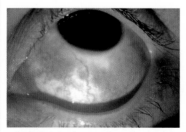

c Oculodermal melanocytosis

B. Surgical changes and trauma

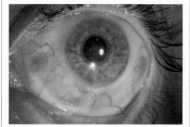

a Scleral atrophy after cyclocryocoagulation

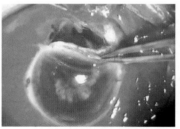

b Traumatic wound dehiscence after cataract extraction at the corneoscleral incision

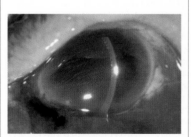

c Rupture of the globe after blunt injury

A. Malformations and Anomalies

Complete absence of the iris is called **aniridia** (**Aa**), though this is usually extreme hypoplasia. Congenital aniridia is bilateral, of autosomal-dominant inheritance (mutations of the PAX6 gene) and often occurs together with other ocular malformations. The rarer sporadic aniridia can be associated with Wilms tumor (more rarely testicular tumors), mental retardation, and malformations of the urogenital tract (**Miller syndrome**). The syndrome is due to mutations and major deletions of the short arm of chromosome 11, which includes the Wilms tumor gene (WT1) as well as the PAX6 gene. Children with sporadic aniridia must therefore undergo regular pediatric examination. Symptomatic therapy for aniridia includes iris-colored contact lenses or an intraocular iris diaphragm in cataract surgery.

Persistent pupillary membrane (**Ab**) arises from incomplete resolution of the tunica vasculosa lentis and mesodermal tissue of the anterior chamber. The degree is very variable. Dense membranes restricting vision are rare and can be excised.

Corectopia describes a usually bilateral, symmetrical displacement of the pupil (especially upward and outward) and is often associated with other ocular malformations.

Heterochromia is a congenital or acquired difference between the two eyes in the color of the iris. Congenital heterochromia can have different causes: simple heterochromia is an isolated anomaly of unknown origin (the affected side has a lighter iris). Sympathetic heterochromia usually arises because of a birth injury of the cervical sympathetic nerves and results in progressive fading and hypoplasia of the iris on the affected side (often combined with Horner syndrome). In addition, heterochromia occurs in melanosis of the iris as part of congenital ocular (**Ac**) or oculodermal melanosis (Ota's nevus). No primary therapy is available.

Oculodermal melanosis (Ota's nevus) is characterized by unilateral (very rarely bilateral) increased melanocytic pigmentation of the lids, conjunctiva, sclera, iris, ciliary body, and choroid (region of distribution of the first and second divisions of the trigeminal nerve). In the rarer purely ocular melanosis there is no skin involvement. Oculodermal melanosis is more common in black people and Asians and is rare in caucasians. There is an increased risk of malignant degeneration only in caucasians (conjunctival and choroidal melanoma). Secondary glaucoma often occurs in the affected eye. Regular follow-up of these patients is necessary.

Iris bicolor (**Ad**) is a rare, unilateral or bilateral, circumscribed hyperpigmentation or hypopigmentation of the iris and does not require any treatment. This also applies to congenital iris cysts located in the iris stroma or at the margin of the pupil.

Congenital **ectropion uveae** is a rare malformation of the pupillary margin, which occurs due to circumscribed protrusion of the pigment layer of the iris and itself does not require any treatment.

Colobomas can be limited to part of the uveal tract (iris, **Ae**; choroid, **Af**) or can involve the entire uveal tract. Colobomas are tissue defects that are due to defective closure of the optic fissure during embryogenesis (5th–8th week) and therefore occur in the lower nasal quadrant. Iris colobomas may require treatment because of increased sensitivity to glare (operative closure of the iris, iris-colored contact lens). Choroidal colobomas can vary between small defects about the diameter of the disk and large defects involving the entire quadrant. No functioning retina can develop in the region of the choroidal coloboma because of the absence of retinal pigment epithelium. If the macula is not affected, visual acuity is normal. The risk of retinal detachment is markedly increased because of a high tendency to retinal tears at the margin of the choroidal coloboma.

A. Malformations and Anomalies

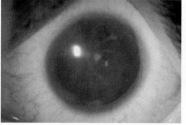

a Aniridia

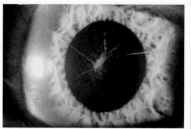

b Persistent pupillary membrane

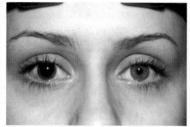

c Ocular melanosis on the right

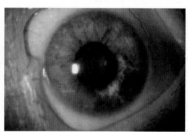

d Iris bicolor

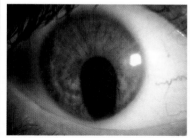

e Iris coloboma

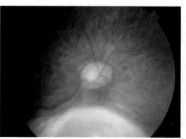

f Retinochoroidal coloboma

A. Dystrophies, Degenerative Conditions, and Age-related Changes

Typical **age-related changes** of the choroid and iris (uveal tract) include atrophy of the pupillary margin, thinning of the iris stroma with atrophy of the sphincter and dilator pupillae muscles, and correspondingly sluggish pupil reaction. Iridoschisis (**Aa**) is rare, where separation of the iris stroma occurs, usually inferiorly. The ciliary body villi and stroma undergo increasing hyalinization in old age. The proportion of connective tissue increases continuously and is accompanied by compensatory hypertrophy of the ciliary muscle, which itself is subject to fibrosis. However, the contractility of the ciliary muscle is preserved throughout life. The atrophic changes also include the ciliary body epithelium. Senile choroidal sclerosis is the name for the increase in the choroidal vascular pattern, which is due particularly to thinning of the retinal pigment epithelium.

Uveal **degeneration** can be a concomitant phenomenon of numerous disease processes with intraocular involvement, including those of a traumatic, inflammatory, postoperative, or ischemic nature. The changes sometimes have a characteristic pattern. Marked degenerative choroidal and retinal changes can be observed especially in severe progressive myopia (**Ab**). The posterior pole including the macula is involved in particular. Oval, round, or geographic zones of atrophy develop in which the retinal pigment epithelium is lacking and the sclera and choroidal vessels become visible.

Dystrophies of the choroid are characterized by progressive destruction of the choriocapillary layer with secondary atrophy of the retinal pigment epithelium (**A, Table 1**).

Central areolar choroid dystrophy usually becomes apparent in the third to fifth decades in the form of exudative, edematous maculopathy. In its subsequent course, symmetrical circumscribed and slowly progressive atrophy of the choroid and retinal pigment epithelium occurs bilaterally in the region of the macula. The loss of function results in a central scotoma. The retinal periphery is not involved.

Gyrate atrophy (**Ac**) is due to a deficiency of the enzyme ornithine ketoaminotransferase (OAT), which leads to raised ornithine concentrations. The disease becomes manifest between the first and second decades. The great majority of patients have high myopia at the same time. The degenerative process begins in the middle retinal periphery and gradually involves the entire retina and choroid. Central visual acuity is preserved for a relatively long time before the process involves the macula. The atrophy at the late stage also extends to the optic disc, retinal vessels, ciliary body, and iris. A secondary cataract can often be observed at this time. Therapeutically, when there is partial OAT function (heterozygosity with 50 % functioning OAT) the activity of the enzyme can be increased by adding the coenzyme vitamin B6 (pyridoxine). The prognosis thus depends substantially on the success of such vitamin supplementation. The ornithine concentration can also be affected by a low-arginine diet or increased renal excretion of arginine.

B. Vascular Changes

Vascular changes in the choroid and iris include hyperemia, hemorrhages, neovascularization, and ischemic conditions. **Rubeosis iridis** (**Ba**) is the term for neovascularization of the iris. The causes are numerous:

- Vascular hypoxia (e.g., central retinal vein occlusion)
- Neoplastic (e.g., choroid melanoma)
- Inflammatory (e.g., uveitis)
- Neuronal/retinal diseases (e.g., diabetic retinopathy)

The rubeosis usually commences at the margin of the pupil and the root of the iris. While the dilated vessels always run radially in pure iris hyperemia, there is irregular, diffuse growth in rubeosis. There is a clearly increased bleeding tendency. Invasion of the anterior chamber angle/trabecular meshwork leads to the development of secondary angle-closure glaucoma due to the formation of anterior synechiae (neovascularization glaucoma, **Bb**).

A. Dystrophies, Degenerative Conditions, and Age-related Changes

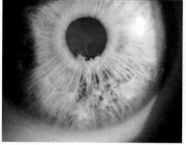

a Iridoschisis

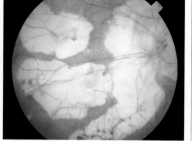

b High myopia

Table 1 Dystrophies of the choroid

Dystrophy	Circumscribed/diffuse	Inheritance
Central areolar choroidal dystrophy	Diffuse	AD
Choroideremia	Diffuse	XR
Gyrate atrophy	Diffuse	AR
Generalized choroidal atrophy	Diffuse	AD, rarely AR
Crystalline retinopathy	Diffuse	AD/AR

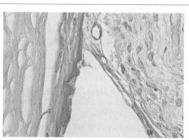

c Gyrate atrophy

Inheritance: AD = autosomal dominant
AR = autosomal recessive
XR = X-linked recessive

B. Vascular Changes

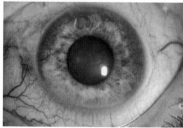

a Rubeosis iridis

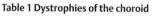

b Peripheral anterior synechiae in neovascular glaucoma (HE stain, 63)

A. Benign Tumors of the Uveal Tract

The most common tumor of the iris is the nevus. Nevi originate from iris melanocytes and usually become visible from around puberty until early adulthood. A distinction is made between circumscribed (**Aa**) and diffuse (**Ab**) iris nevi. Circumscribed nevi can be very varied in position, size, degree of pigmentation, and shape. There is not usually an increase in size. If the nevus located at the pupillary margin, there can be pupil irregularity and ectropion uveae. Diffuse iris nevi are flatter and involve an entire sector or even the entire iris. The diagnosis is made clinically and should be confirmed by monitoring progress. Malignant transformation is rare.

Iris pigment epithelial cysts (Ac) are usually idiopathic in nature; more rarely, they occur after medical therapy (e.g., miotics). There is an increased incidence in middle age. They are brownish, roundish tumors at the pupillary margin or in the center of the iris stroma. When they are located peripherally they are not visible directly and are apparent because of protrusion of the iris stroma. The diagnosis is made on the basis of the clinical picture and with ultrasonic biomicroscopy. No treatment necessary.

Varix nodes of the iris are very rare, convexly rounded, brown-black tumors with a clear tendency to bleeding. There is usually spontaneous regression.

Primary benign tumors of the ciliary body are rare (leiomyomas, adenomas, cysts). The **medulloepithelioma of the ciliary body** usually becomes apparent in childhood as a unilateral, unifocal tumor of the ciliary body. Benign and malignant forms are distinguished. Extraocular growth and metastasis are possible. With locally limited growth, treatment is block excision of the tumor, otherwise enucleation.

Nevi of the choroid (Ad) are the most common intraocular tumors. The etiology is unclear. They are located mainly at the posterior pole and are quite often multifocal or bilateral. In the great majority of cases they remain asymptomatic. Approximately 90% of the nevi are between 0.5 and 6 mm in size. Clinically they are round to oval grayish brown lesions, with their edges not completely demarcated and without significant height (< 1 mm). In contrast to choroidal melanoma, the nevus usually disappears in light free of red wavelengths. Up to 50% of the nevi have drusen on the surface as an expression of a chronic stationary process. Treatment is required only rarely. Malignant transformation occurs in about 1 : 5000 per year.

Hemangiomas of the choroid (Ae) are rare. Diffuse and circumscribed forms are distinguished. The diffuse hemangiomas are usually associated with Sturge-Weber syndrome and often infiltrate more than half of the entire uveal tract. They are diagnosed within the first decade. The localized hemangiomas usually become symptomatic only around the fourth or fifth decades and are located mainly at the posterior pole. Clinically the appearance of choroidal hemangiomas is of a reddish-orange color. There is no tendency to growth. Independent of the form, they lead in up to 80% to exudative retinal detachment and retinal degeneration. Secondary glaucoma can be expected particularly with the diffuse hemangioma. Asymptomatic hemangiomas do not require any treatment. If there are complications, laser coagulation or photodynamic therapy can be used.

Choroidal osteoma (Af) is an ossified lesion occurring in the second to third decade, mainly in women. It is bilateral in about 25%. A juxtapapillary, well-demarcated, irregular whitish yellow elevation is characteristic. The diagnosis is confirmed by echography (maximum reflectivity). Histologically mature bone tissue with medullary spaces is seen. No treatment available.

Bilateral uveal hyperplasia is very rare and is characterized by an increasing number of bilateral, nevuslike choroidal lesions. Ocular complications occur rapidly (cataract, uveitis, retinal detachment). The lesions probably consist of uveal melanocytes, which are stimulated to proliferation by growth factors from malignant tumors. The uveal changes precede the actual tumor manifestation by months. The primary tumors are tumors of the gastrointestinal tract, the lung, and the female reproductive organs. The search for and treatment of the primary tumor take priority.

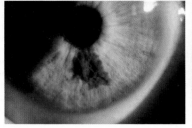

a Circumscribed iris nevus

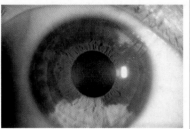

b Diffuse iris nevus

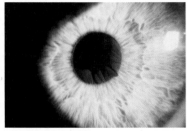

c Iris pigment epithelial cysts

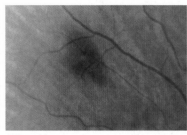

d Choroidal nevus

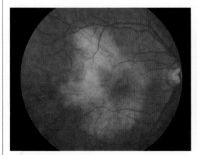

e Choroidal hemangioma

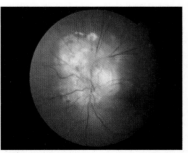

f Choroidal osteoma

A. Malignant Melanoma of the Iris and Ciliary Body

The malignant tumors of the uveal tract are predominantly malignant melanoma and metastases from primary extraocular tumors.

Etiology/pathogenesis. Unknown.

Epidemiology. Malignant melanomas of the iris account for about 3–10% and ciliary body melanomas for about 9% of all uveal melanomas. Both forms are rare overall.

Clinical features. Circumscribed **iris melanomas** are distinguished clinically from diffuse ones (**Aa**). In both cases feeder vessels from the circulus arteriosus iridis major are often found. The degree of pigmentation of the tumor can be very variable. With the more frequent circumscribed tumors, distinction from an iris nevus is usually possible only by a proven tendency to growth. Prominence of the tumor, corneal edema, and incipient bands of corneal degeneration often indicate an active growth process clinically. Diffuse iris melanomas are rarer and often become apparent because of the combination of heterochromia (affected side darker) and increased intraocular pressure. Clinically the thickened, faded, or often darker iris surface and a more pigmented chamber angle are apparent when the sides are compared.

The ciliary body melanoma (**Ab–e**) is often only discovered late because of its location. Usually rather nonspecific symptoms such as localized cataract, pigment dispersion with or without secondary glaucoma, vitreous hemorrhage, retinal detachment, circumscribed episcleritis, or uveitis lead to the diagnosis. Besides localized tumors, annular diffuse growth (ring melanoma) with early invasion of the chamber angle ("unilateral pigment glaucoma") can occur very rarely, where the tumor can only be demonstrated with difficulty and therefore is often diagnosed late.

Diagnosis. With iris melanomas, extension of the tumor in the posterior direction must be excluded. With ciliary body melanoma, fine-needle biopsy may be required to detect the tumor. To exclude an extraocular primary tumor/metastasis, a chest radiograph, abdominal ultrasound, and dermatological and urological or gynecological investigations should be performed.

Differential diagnosis. Iris nevus.

Treatment. If there is a clear tendency to growth, the treatment of circumscribed iris melanomas usually consists of a primary globe-preserving surgical procedure (iridectomy, iridocyclectomy). If excision is successful, the prognosis for vision is often good. Treatment of diffuse iris melanomas, which are associated with a much worse prognosis for vision because of the secondary glaucoma, is much more difficult and often leads to enucleation in the advanced stage. This also applies for the diffuse form of ciliary body melanoma.

Prognosis. The prognosis in terms of survival is good for iris melanomas, and metastasis is very rare. Ciliary body melanomas, like all uveal melanomas, have a poor prognosis because they are diagnosed late.

B. Metastases of the Iris and Ciliary Body

Iris metastases are rare and account for about 5–10% of all ocular metastases. There is often involvement of the ciliary body at the same time. They arise as a result of hematogenous metastasis from extraocular tumors. Elderly patients are mainly affected. The primary tumors are especially breast (**B**) and lung cancer, more rarely cutaneous melanoma, gastrointestinal carcinoma, and bronchial carcinoids.

Clinically, a whitish or flesh-colored tumor (pigmentation in the case of metastatic melanoma) with an irregular surface can be observed. Usually unilocular, occasionally multilocular, rarely bilateral, ipsilateral or contralateral metastasis to the choroid at the same time in about one-third. The suspected diagnosis is made clinically; usually the primary tumor is already known. The differential diagnosis includes amelanotic melanoma, granulomas, xanthogranulomas, or leiomyomas. Treatment of the primary tumor is primary treatment (with interdisciplinary collaboration); local external radiation or brachytherapy are also possible, more rarely surgical excision of the metastasis.

A. Malignant Melanoma of the Iris and Ciliary Body

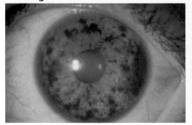

a Iris melanoma

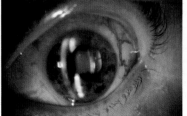

b Ciliary body melanoma

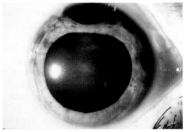

c Ciliary body melanoma penetrating anteriorly

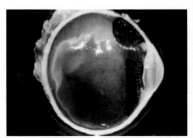

d Macroscopic appearance of a ciliary body melanoma

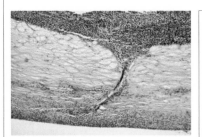

e Penetration of a ciliary body melanoma through the sclera along an emissary vein

B. Metastases of Iris and Ciliary Body

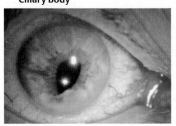

Metastasis from a breast cancer

A. Malignant Melanoma of the Choroid

Malignant melanoma of the choroid is the most common primary malignant intraocular tumor.

Etiology/pathogenesis. Unclear.

Epidemiology. Incidence of uveal melanoma is about 6 per 1 million population per year. Of these, 80–90% are melanomas of the choroid. Peak incidence is in the sixth and seventh decades.

Clinical features. The symptoms are a reduction in vision and visual field, more rarely changes in the iris and pupil following tumor extension into the anterior chamber. Clinical examination shows a usually unilocular tumor, mainly in the region of the posterior uveal tract. Occasionally there is increased episcleral vascular filling over the tumor ("sentinel vessels"). The tumor has a smooth surface with a brown, gray, or black color (white in the case of amelanotic melanoma). Superficial deposits of lipofuscin ("orange pigment", **Aa**), tumor-induced, exudative detachment at the lower edge of the tumor, and a mushroom tumor shape (**Ab** and **c**) are highly suggestive of melanoma. With necrotic melanomas, intraocular inflammation is frequent (about 5% of all choroidal melanomas appear initially as inflammation). Occasionally secondary glaucoma with rubeosis iridis or direct chamber angle invasion are seen. Choroidal melanomas grow slowly with a tumor doubling time of about 30 days (epithelioid cell melanoma, **Ad**) to 350 days (spindle cell melanoma).

Diagnosis. The diagnosis is made from the clinical appearance, echography, and diaphanoscopy, and possibly fine-needle biopsy. Exclusion of a primary extraocular tumor/metastasis by chest radiography (or thoracic CT), upper abdominal ultrasound, consultation with dermatology, gynecology, urology (whole-body MRI if necessary).

Differential diagnosis. Choroidal nevus and metastases, disciform macular degeneration, choroidal hemorrhage and detachment, hypertrophy of the retinal pigment epithelium, hamartomas.

Treatment. Depends on the patient's age and general condition, tumor size and location, and accompanying ocular changes. A range of therapeutic options is available: observation without intervention; local radiotherapy through applicators (brachytherapy); direct destruction of the tumor tissue by laser energy (transpupillary thermotherapy [TTT]); endoresection of the tumor; transscleral tumor resection and enucleation. Overall, there is a trend toward primary globe-preserving procedures.

Prognosis. The mortality rate remains the same across the different forms of therapy. About 40% of patients develop liver metastases within 10 years after the diagnosis is made. The mean survival time after liver metastases have occurred is between 2 and 7 months. Prognostic parameters for the development of metastases are tumor location (especially ciliary body involvement), tumor size (greatest tumor diameter), histological cell type (epithelioid cells), tumor invasion (deep sclera, extraocular growth), and certain vessel patterns and monosomy 3 in the tumor.

B. Metastases of the Choroid

Metastases are the most common intraocular malignancies overall and about 80–90% of them are located in the choroid. They occur mainly at a later age as a result of hematogenous metastasis of extraocular tumors. Most of them are carcinomas, especially **breast cancer** (**Ba**, 40–50% overall) and **lung cancer** (**Bb**, 20–30%), more rarely tumors of the gastrointestinal tract or kidney, or carcinoids. Of the nonepithelial tumors, malignant cutaneous melanoma is the most common tumor metastasizing to the choroid.

Most choroidal metastases are located at the posterior pole. The main symptom is painless deterioration of vision. The clinical picture is characterized by unilocular or multilocular, yellowish, grayish or gray-red infiltrations, which are not very elevated. There is often an accompanying exudative retinal detachment.

The treatment of the primary tumor is also the treatment of the choroidal metastases (chemotherapy or hormone therapy). This, along with adjuvant local irradiation, often produces regression of the ocular metastases. The prognosis with regard to life expectancy is poor because of generalized tumor spread.

A. Malignant Melanoma of the Choroid

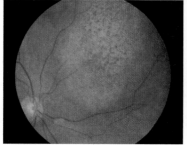

a Choroidal melanoma with orange pigment

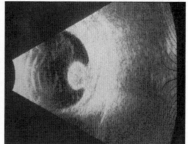

b Ultrasound appearance of a choroidal melanoma with typical mushroom shape

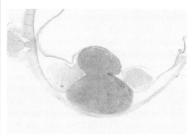

c Choroidal melanoma with "collar-stud" appearance on penetration of Bruch's membrane

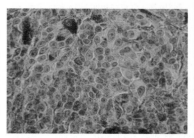

d Histology of an epithelioid cell type of choroidal melanoma

B. Metastases of the Choroid

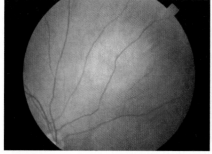

a Multilocular metastases from breast cancer

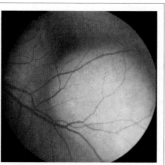

b Metastasis from a bronchial carcinoma

A. Surgical Changes

The well-perfused uveal tract is always subject to a particular risk of bleeding during surgery and has a tendency to inflammatory conditions. An alteration of the iris, e. g., after cataract surgery, can lead rapidly to the development of a **fibrin reaction of the anterior chamber**, and wide panlaser coagulation of the retina can lead to **consecutive choroidal swelling**. The **choroidal effusion syndrome** is a very rare complication, where massive bleeding into the choroid can be triggered by a relatively sudden drop in intraocular pressure. Occasionally, particularly after pressure-lowering procedures, **choroidal detachment** (**A**), which is due to the low intraocular pressure, occurs postoperatively and resolves spontaneously when the intraocular pressure rises again.

B. Changes in the Uveal Tract with Penetrating Injuries

Penetrating injuries of the eye are open-eye injuries that are caused by the penetration of pointed or sharp objects into the eye. Younger men and children are mainly affected. The uveal tract is nearly always involved. There can be a direct tear of uveal tissue, or it can be damaged by prolapsing into the wound gap (**B**). The diagnosis is usually straightforward. When the history warrants, imaging procedures should be performed to visualize intraocular foreign bodies. The primary management is watertight closure of the wound. In the further management, correction of tissue defects (e. g., pupillary defect due to a tear of the iris) can be performed. Sympathetic ophthalmia is one of the late complications (see below).

C. Contusion of the Globe

Contusion of the globe describes a contusion of the eye due to the effect of blunt force.

Etiology/pathogenesis. The injuries are due to:
- Compression of the anterior segment of the eye with expansion of the eyeball equator
- The expansion phase following the compression phase with longitudinal stretching of the globe (injuries of the posterior segment of the eye)
- Propagation of the contusion wave (coup-contrecoup effect)

With extreme compression forces exceeding the resistance of the wall of the eyeball, rupture of the globe occurs, often with prolapse of uveal tissue.

Epidemiology. 1–7% of all ocular injuries. Mainly younger men (> 80%).

Clinical features. A number of ocular structures can be affected with a variable degree of severity. Frequent nonuveal changes are lid edema or hematoma, subconjunctival hemorrhage, cataract, and Berlin's edema of the retina. The uveal changes include iritis (100%), anterior chamber angle recession (50–80%), tear of the root of the iris (iridodialysis, 4–30%, **Ca**), hyphema (50–60%, **Cb**), mydriasis (up to 50%), and rarely tears of the iris sphincter (**Cc**), cyclodialysis, choroidal hemorrhage, choroidal rupture (**Cd**), chorioretinitis sclopetaria (rupture of the retina and choroid), and subsequent choroidal atrophy.

Diagnosis. The diagnosis is made from the clinical appearance. CT is used if globe rupture or orbital fracture is suspected.

Differential diagnosis. Closed-globe rupture, penetrating injury with or without intraocular foreign body.

Treatment. Globe contusion is treated conservatively: physical rest, no reading, local corticosteroids depending on the degree of inflammation, and pressure-lowering medications as needed. If an anterior chamber hemorrhage fails to reabsorb, a hematocornea develops, or the rise in intraocular pressure cannot be controlled medically, surgical removal of the hyphema is performed. Operative closure should be performed if the globe is ruptured.

Prognosis. There is usually a very good prognosis for vision. The prevalence of traumatic secondary glaucoma is about 0.5–9%. The vision prognosis is much worse if there is a choroidal rupture at the posterior pole, globe rupture, hemophthalmos, retinal detachment, or traumatic optic neuropathy.

A. Surgical Changes

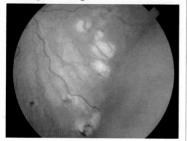

Choroidal detachment

B. Penetrating Injuries

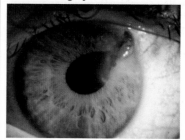

Corneal wound with iris prolapse

C. Blunt Ocular Trauma (Contusion)

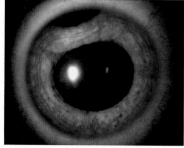

a Iris dialysis

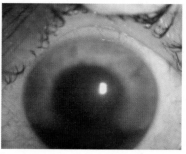

b Hyphema

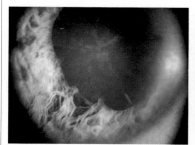

c Iris sphincter defect and traumatic rosette cataract

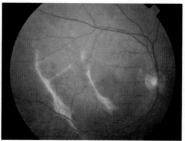

d Choroidal rupture

A. Definition and classification of uveal inflammation

Uveitis is the term for primary inflammation of the uveal tract of various causes. From the anatomical aspect, differentiation is made into:
- Anterior uveitis: iritis, iridocyclitis
- Intermediate uveitis
- Posterior uveitis: choroiditis, chorioretinitis, retinochoroiditis
- Panuveitis: anterior and posterior uveitis

The course can be acute, acute-recurrent, or chronic (inflammation persisting longer than three months). With regard to the etiology, infectious, traumatic, iatrogenic (postoperative, drug-related), immunologically mediated (with or without systemic disease), and idiopathic forms can be distinguished.

B. Anterior Uveitis

Anterior uveitis is inflammation that is limited to the iris (iritis) or to the iris and ciliary body (iridocyclitis).

Etiology/pathogenesis. The most common causes of infectious anterior uveitis in Western Europe are borreliosis, tuberculosis, syphilis, and herpes viruses. A large proportion is non-infectious and can be interpreted as a primary autoimmune event (**B, Table 1**). In 40–60% of the acute forms there is an association with HLA–B27. Traumatic origins may follow contusion, intraocular injuries, and surgery; it is rarely due to medications or contact lenses.

Epidemiology. The most common form of uveitis (ca. 60%). An incidence of 17/100 000 and prevalence of 34/100 000 are assumed for all forms of uveitis.

Clinical features. Acute anterior uveitis is characterized by sudden onset with pain, red eye, epiphora, sensitivity to glare, and deterioration of vision. Mixed injection (conjunctival and ciliary, **Ba**), deposits on the back of the cornea (**Bb**), severe inflammation of the anterior chamber (cells, Tyndall phenomenon) ranging up to a fibrin reaction, inflammatory miosis, and adhesions between the iris and lens are often found. Particularly severe disease is associated with hypopyon (a deposit of leukocytes on the floor of the anterior chamber). Chronic anterior uveitis (**Bc**) has a slowly progressive course with an externally noninflamed eye. There is no pain, so that deterioration in vision is noticed as the main symptom. Because of the initially slight symptoms, the diagnosis is often made late, especially in children with juvenile idiopathic arthritis. When the course is prolonged, secondary changes then occur, such as bandlike corneal degeneration (Bd), secondary cataract (posterior subcapsular cataract), and secondary glaucoma.

Diagnosis. A careful general history is required since anterior uveitis is often a concomitant phenomenon with systemic diseases. Sometimes a typical clinical picture (heterochromic cyclitis, herpes simplex keratouveitis) leads directly to the diagnosis. When examining the patient, particular attention should be paid to complications of anterior uveitis (macular edema, cataract, glaucoma). Chest radiography to exclude active tuberculosis and sarcoidosis. Serological exclusion of syphilis and borreliosis. In addition, angiotensin-converting enzyme (ACE) as a marker of sarcoidosis and possibly HLA–B27 in acute-recurrent anterior uveitis. In the case of general symptoms, investigation should always be demanded. In children, look for antinuclear antibodies (ANA) and perform pediatric rheumatology investigation for juvenile idiopathic arthritis.

Differential diagnosis. Old retinal detachment, pigment dispersion syndrome, intraocular hemorrhage, endophthalmitis.

Treatment. With infectious origin, appropriate treatment with antiviral agents or antibiotics (e.g., in borreliosis). Noninfectious uveitis is treated symptomatically. Local therapy consists of corticosteroid eye drops and mydriatics/cycloplegics to avoid posterior synechiae between the iris and lens and to suppress pain by resting the ciliary body. If necessary, supplement with subconjunctival, parabulbar, or oral administration of corticosteroids. Immunosuppression is rarely needed in chronic or frequently recurring uveitis.

B. Anterior Uveitis

Table 1 Systemic diseases in anterior uveitis

Joints	Seronegative spondylarthropathies Juvenile idiopathic arthritis
Connective tissue	Systemic lupus erythematosus Recurrent polychondritis Dermatomyositis
Vasculitis	Behçet disease Polyarteritis nodosa Wegener granulomatosis Cogan syndrome II
Infectious/granulomatous	Syphilis Tuberculosis Borreliosis Leprosy Herpes simplex Sarcoidosis
Intestine	Ulcerative colitis Crohn disease
Kidney	tubulointerstitial nephritis and uveitis (TINU) syndrome
Skin	Ophthalmic zoster

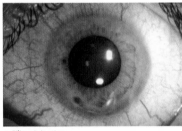

a Ciliary injection

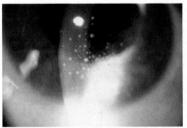

b Large keratic precipitates ("greasy" appearing deposits on the corneal endothelium) in the lower half of the cornea

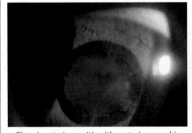

c Chronic anterior uveitis with posterior synechiae and secondary cataract

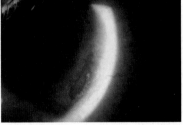

d Bandlike corneal degeneration

A. Herpes Simplex Keratouveitis

The acute-recurrent keratouveitis caused by re-activation of HSV-1 is characterized by decreased corneal sensitivity, keratitis (often pre-existing corneal stromal scarring with neovascularization, **A**), anterior chamber inflammation, adhesions between the iris and lens, and diffuse iris pigment epithelium defects. Secondary cataract and glaucoma (trabeculitis) are common. Local anti-inflammatory and antiviral therapy and systemic antiviral therapy for a prolonged period is required and also to prevent recurrence.

B. Heterochromic Iridocyclitis (Fuchs)

Fuchs heterochromic cyclitis is a rare, chronic iridocyclitis of unknown origin, unilateral in 90%, without ethnic, age, or sex predilection. There are usually few symptoms, but occasionally there is recurrent anterior chamber hemorrhage. In its classical form, it is characterized by an externally uninflamed eye; heterochromia (affected eye lighter, **Ba**); fine, sometimes stellate posterior deposits distributed diffusely over the entire corneal endothelium; moderate anterior chamber inflammation; iris stromal atrophy (**Bb**); absence of adhesions between the iris and lens; secondary cataract (posterior capsule opacity); and cellular infiltration of the severely degenerative vitreous body. There are frequently vascular anomalies in the anterior chamber angle. There is no retinal involvement. It is usually mild, so that treatment is not necessary. Moreover, the inflammation is hardly affected by corticosteroids. The main problem is the development of secondary glaucoma in 5–60% of all patients, which is difficult to treat.

C. Intermediate Uveitis

Intermediate uveitis is the term for intraocular inflammation characterized by inflammatory changes in the vitreous body, retinal vascular sheathing, and/or predominant infiltration of the pars plana of the ciliary body (pars planitis). Infiltration of the choroid is not a feature of the disease (cf. posterior uveitis).

Etiology/pathogenesis. The etiology usually remains unclear. Known causes are borreliosis, syphilis, sarcoidosis. Association with disseminated encephalomyelitis.

Epidemiology. 5–20% of all uveitides, one-third of pediatric uveitides. Bilateral in 70–90%.

Clinical features. The main symptom is painless deterioration of vision (blurred vision, floaters). It is often an incidental finding as the eye may not be inflamed externally. Visual acuity varies depending on the degree of inflammation. Anterior chamber inflammation can be present. There are usually numerous cells in the vitreous body, and the vitreous body skeleton/framework often also has a streaky appearance (**Ca, b**). There may be whitish, fluffy to sharply demarcated accumulations of inflammatory cells ("snowballs", **Cc**) peripherally, mainly in the lower circumference. In pars planitis the changes can be limited to dense whitish membranes ("snowbanks") lying on the pars plana. There is often inflammatory sheathing, particularly of venous vessels and especially peripherally. There are often complications such as macular edema, secondary cataract, and secondary glaucoma with chronic persistent inflammation. There is risk of hemorrhage and development of holes with retinal detachment through contraction of the vitreous body.

Diagnosis. The diagnosis is made clinically. Borreliosis, syphilis, and sarcoidosis should be excluded (serology, chest radiography). Neurological investigation is called for with symptoms of disseminated encephalomyelitis.

Differential diagnosis. Endophthalmitis, masquerade syndrome (intraocular lymphoma, old retinal detachment).

Treatment. Antibiotics when the origin is infectious. Monitoring without therapy in idiopathic cases with good visual acuity, low inflammatory activity, and absence of complications. With slight inflammatory activity, possibly parabulbar corticosteroid administration. More severe inflammation with macular edema requires systemic therapy with oral corticosteroids (initially 1–2 mg prednisolone equivalent/kg/day); in macular edema this might be combined with carbonic anhydrase inhibitors (acetazolamide). Immunosuppression additionally in severe disease (e.g., cyclosporine A).

Prognosis. Mainly good prognosis for vision.

A. Herpes Simplex Keratouveitis

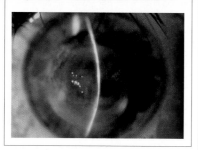

C. Intermediate Uveitis

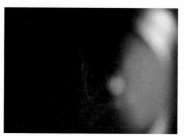

a Cellular infiltration of the anterior vitreous body

B. Heterochromic Cyclitis

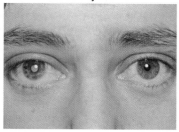

a Heterochromia and cataract in the right eye

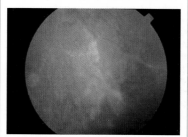

b Retinal vascular sheathing and vitreous membranes

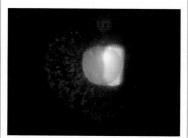

b Retroillumination of the iris with diffuse defects of the iris pigment epithelium

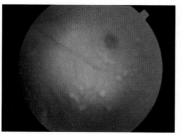

c "Snowballs" in the vitreous body

A. Posterior Uveitis

Posterior uveitis is a blanket term for a heterogeneous group of diseases that are associated primarily with inflammatory changes of the choroid (often with secondary involvement of the retina).

Etiology/pathogenesis. Very heterogeneous and unclarified in many respects (T cell-mediated reaction to uveal antigens; direct inflammatory reaction to pathogens that have migrated into the uveal tract). Infectious causes (e.g., tuberculosis), autoimmune diseases (e.g., Cogan syndrome), or idiopathic causes are possible (**A, Table 1**).

Epidemiology. Approximately 20% of all uveitides. Most commonly due to toxoplasmosis or sarcoidosis (**Aa**).

Clinical features. Nearly always deterioration in vision. Distorted vision, with and without pain or red eye. Often severe inflammatory changes in the vitreous body, which can prevent a view of the retina and choroid. Vasculitis of retinal vessels is possible. Involvement of the choroid in the form of individual or multiple inflammatory lesions (**Ab**). Characteristic changes in individual diseases at times, which allow diagnosis.

Diagnosis. With the typical clinical picture (e.g., toxoplasmosis), no further investigations are required. Otherwise chest radiography to exclude sarcoidosis/tuberculosis; serology for borreliosis, syphilis, angiotensin-converting enzyme, toxocariasis in childhood. Further interdisciplinary investigation if systemic disease is suspected. Aspiration of vitreous body when the course is resistant to treatment.

Differential diagnosis. Masquerade syndrome (old retinal detachment, intraocular lymphoma), endophthalmitis.

Treatment. With infectious cause, treatment is primarily curative and anti-infectious. With idiopathic or autoimmune disease, treatment is symptomatic, usually with oral corticosteroids (initially 1–2 mg prednisolone equivalent/kg/day). Immunosuppression should be given if necessary in severe disease.

Prognosis. Depends on the underlying disease and severity of the disease.

B. Toxoplasmosis Retinochoroiditis

Toxoplasmosis retinochoroiditis is the most common form of posterior uveitis.

Etiology/pathogenesis. The disease is caused by infection with the protozoon Toxoplasma gondii. Intrauterine infection can occur if the mother is infected during pregnancy (congenital toxoplasmosis) or infection can occur postnatally (acquired toxoplasmosis).

Epidemiology. Serological evidence of prior toxoplasmosis has a high prevalence and 70–90% of cases of congenital toxoplasmosis and about 2–4% with acquired toxoplasmosis develop toxoplasmosis retinochoroiditis. Immunosuppressed and HIV patients have a markedly increased risk of toxoplasmosis.

Clinical features. The primary intrauterine infection usually passes unnoticed (subclinical). Recurrences of congenital toxoplasmosis often lead to bilateral (30%) chorioretinal scarring (**Ba, b**) with a preference for the posterior pole, including the macula. Late ocular damage develops due to further recurrences of the retinochoroiditis, which originates in the marginal area of scars that are already present. Other ocular manifestations are anterior chamber inflammation, retinal vasculitis, papillitis (Jensen's juxtapapillary retinitis) and neuroophthalmological manifestations with CNS infection.

Diagnosis. With a good view of the fundus, retinochoroiditis is diagnosed clinically because of the typical appearance.

Differential diagnosis. With a poor view of the fundus, all other forms of posterior uveitis, panuveitis, endophthalmitis.

Treatment. Treatment is with a combination of corticosteroids and pyrimethamine/sulfadiazine combination or clindamycin when there is a chorioretinal infiltrate within the large vascular arcades with involvement of or a threat to the macula or massive vitreous infiltration. It is not curative and serves primarily to protect ocular structures. Peripheral infiltrates can be observed in immunocompetent patients.

Prognosis. The active stage is self-limiting. The prognosis for vision is generally good, depending on the location. Recurrences are possible at any time.

A. Posterior Uveitis

Table 1 Differential diagnosis of posterior uveitis

Idiopathic	Serpiginous chorioretinitis Multifocal chorioretinitis White dot syndrome (APMPPE, MEWDS, and others).
Granulomatous	Sarcoidosis
Infectious diseases	Histoplasmosis Tuberculosis Syphilis Borreliosis Toxoplasmosis Toxocariasis
Autoimmune diseases/vasculitis	Behçet disease Cogan syndrome II Vogt-Koyanagi–Harada syndrome

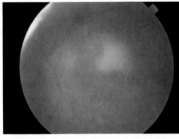

a Central choroidal granuloma in sarcoidosis

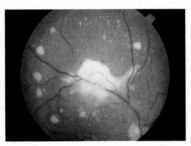

b Multifocal choroiditis

B. Toxoplasmosis Retinochoroiditis

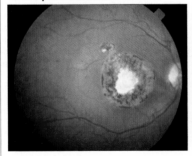

a Typical central scarring

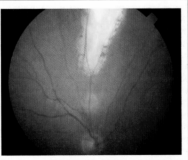

b Large choroidal scar with old pigmentation above and new infiltrate below

A. Serpiginous (Geographic) Chorioretinopathy

Serpiginous chorioretinopathy is a rare bilateral, asymmetric to symmetric, slowly progressive disease that leads to gradual loss of the retinal pigment epithelium and the choriocapillary layer.

Etiology/pathogenesis. Unknown.

Epidemiology. Whites in the fouthth to sixth decades are affected predominantly. Clinical features. The course is variable and years can pass between individual periods of activity. The clinical picture is characterized initially by peripapillary infiltrates and scarring, from which there is finger-shaped spread in the direction of the macula (**Aa**). Isolated foci can occur at the posterior pole as far as the middle of the periphery.

Diagnosis. Diagnosis is made from the clinical appearance and fluorescence angiography (**Ab, c**). On fluorescence angiography, fresh foci typically show early block and late hyperfluorescence.

Differential diagnosis. Posterior uveitis from other causes.

Treatment. Systemic therapy with corticosteroids alone cannot usually control the disease activity sufficiently. Early systemic immunosuppression (cyclosporin A, alkylating agents) is therefore recommended.

Prognosis. Because of the progressive scarring of the macula and frequent macular choroidal neovascularization, the prognosis for vision is poor if not treated. The prognosis appears to be better with immunosuppressant treatment.

B. Panuveitis

Panuveitis is the term for simultaneous anterior and posterior uveitis (**B**). However, panuveitis is rare overall and can be due to infection (borreliosis), granulomatous disease (sarcoidosis), or autoimmune disease (sympathetic ophthalmia), or can form part of severe immunological systemic diseases (Behçet disease, Vogt-Koyanagi-Harada syndrome). Curative treatment is given in the case of an infectious cause and the treatment is symptomatic when the cause is idiopathic or immunological (see treatment of anterior and posterior uveitis on pp. 126 and 130). The prognosis for vision depends on the disease in each case, but is often poor.

C. Sympathetic Ophthalmia

Sympathetic ophthalmia is a bilateral, granulomatous panuveitis that classically occurs following a penetrating injury of the eye with uveal involvement. It can also result from ocular surgery.

Etiology/pathogenesis. T cell-mediated autoimmune reaction, caused by release of uveal antigens (probably from melanocytes). Genetic predisposition (association with HLA-DRB1*04 and DQA1*03).

Epidemiology. Very rare. Manifestation may be days to many years after the causative trauma (90% within one year).

Clinical features. The visual acuity is variable. Greasy-appearing deposits on the back of the cornea, variable anterior chamber inflammation, inflammatory cells in the vitreous. Choroidal thickening, papillitis, retinal vascular sheathing, Fuchs-Dalen nodules (small white infiltrates in the middle periphery of the fundus) (**C**). Macular edema, exudative retinal detachment, and optic atrophy are also possible.

Diagnosis. Diagnosis is made clinically when panuveitis from other causes is excluded.

Differential diagnosis. Endophthalmitis, other forms of panuveitis, masquerade syndromes (intraocular lymphoma).

Treatment. There is high risk of blindness without adequate treatment if bilateral. Administration of local and systemic corticosteroids constitutes the basic therapy. Use of immunosuppressants (e.g. cyclosporine A) is often also required.

Prognosis. Recurrences are frequent following reduction or cessation of therapy. Long-term or even lifetime treatment is therefore necessary. The most common complications interfering with vision are macular edema, secondary cataract, and secondary glaucoma.

A. Serpiginous Chorioretinopathy

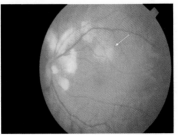

a Active lesion (arrow) adjacent to scarred areas

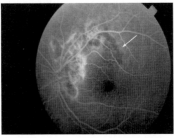

b Fluorescence angiography in the early phase

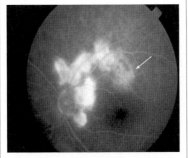

c Fluorescence angiography: diffuse leakage (arrow) in the late phase

B. Panuveitis

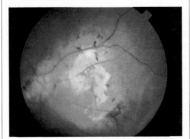

Panuveitis due to tuberculosis

C. Sympathetic Ophthalmia

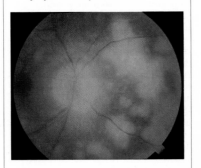

The crystalline lens, along with the vitreous body, is the most centrally located structure of the eye and forms a functional unit with the zonular apparatus and the ciliary body. Compared to the cornea, it has a much lower **converging power** of ca. 17 diopters because of the relatively similar refractive indices of aqueous humor, lens, and vitreous body (cornea ca. 42 D). However, the lens is the only part of the refractive apparatus that is adjustable. Adjustment to near vision (accommodation) therefore involves only the lens. In addition, the lens functions as a **UV filter** for wavelengths between 300 and 400 nm and thus has a protective function for the macula.

The lens reacts to harmful influences in a limited fashion and may display opacification (cataract) and discoloration, restriction of accommodation, and displacement (subluxation or dislocation).

A. Malformations and Anomalies

A genuine fissure of the lens (coloboma) occurs rarely. However, fissures of the uveal tract can be associated with a coloboma of the zonular fibers (**Aa**) and then lead to notching of the lens (**"pseudocoloboma"**) due to the lack of tension in this region.

Deviations from the normal lens shape include a **spherical lens** (**spherophakia, Ab**) and **lenticonus** or lentiglobus, in which the lens "bulges out" in front or behind. **Spherophakia** can cause glaucoma by occluding the pupil, while lenticonus and lentiglobus usually remain asymptomatic, especially when they are mild.

Congenital absence of the lens (**congenital aphakia**) in an otherwise normal and functioning eye has not been observed hitherto. Probably the lens functions as an inducer for further eye development, so that absence of the lens is not compatible with normal eye development. Lens duplication (biphakia) is very unusual.

The congenital lens opacities, which can be interpreted as malformations, are discussed below.

B. Deposits on the Lens and Intralenticular Deposits

Remnants of the pupillary membrane (**persistent pupillary membrane**) can lie on the anterior lens surface as pigment cells or as strands of connective tissue arising from the iris collarette (**Ba**). They are only rarely of clinical significance. With increasing age, deposits of **pseudoexfoliation material** (**PEX; Bb**) may occur. These often become visible only when the pupil is dilated and predispose to glaucoma and lens subluxation (q. v.).

Intraocular foreign bodies of iron can cause rusting of the lens (**siderosis lentis**, see below), while corresponding copper foreign bodies or Wilson disease can induce a yellow-green discoloration of the lens (chalcosis lentis) also known as **sunflower cataract**. Granular gold deposits located under the lens (chrysiasis lentis) can occasionally occur after prolonged treatment with gold preparations (e. g. in primary chronic polyarthritis [PCP]). Other **medications**, e. g., amiodarone or chlorpromazine, are sometimes deposited in the lens. In patients with cataract, glittering cholesterol crystals are not infrequently found in the lens (so-called **Christmas tree decoration cataract, Bc**). However, there does not appear to be an association with blood lipid levels.

A. Malformations and Anomalies

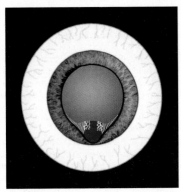

a Iris-zonule coloboma (diagram): retraction of the lens in the region of the zonular defect ("pseudo lens coloboma")

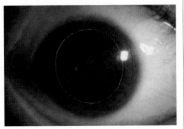

b Spherical lens (spherophakia) in homocystinuria; the lens equator is visible at the edge of the pupil; risk of pupillary block glaucoma

B. Deposits on the Lens and Intralenticular Deposits

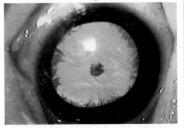

a Remnants of the pupillary membrane (persistent pupillary membrane) on the anterior surface of the lens in a baby; typically, the connective tissue strands attach not at the margin of the pupil but at the iris collarette

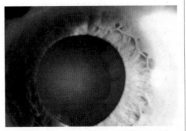

b Deposits of pseudoexfoliation (PEX) material on the lens; the anterior pole of the lens is usually spared

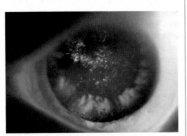

c Cholesterol crystals in an opacified lens (Christmas tree cataract)

A. Presbyopia

Presbyopia (impairment of vision due to old age) is present when the accommodation ability of the lens is no longer sufficient to enable sharp and comfortable near vision.

Etiology/pathogenesis. The mechanisms of **accommodation** and the changes that lead to presbyopia have not been fully elucidated. Current theories of accommodation assume that the ciliary muscle is relaxed when looking into the distance (disaccommodation), so that the zonular fibers are tensed and the lens adopts a flatter shape (with lower converging power). During accommodation there is contraction of the parasympathetically innervated ciliary muscle, which is composed of different muscle portions, and it protrudes inward as a result. This relieves the zonular fibers so that the lens can deform (become thicker) because of its innate elasticity, with the curvature of the posterior lens surface increasing in particular (**Aa**). The now more spherical lens has greater converging power and thus allows sharp near vision. On looking into the distance again, the lens again adopts the flat disaccommodated shape through slackening of the ciliary muscle and tension of the zonular fibers (**Aa**).

With increasing age, the elasticity of the lens diminishes as a result of the continuing appositional growth of lens fibers. The contractility of the ciliary muscle also diminishes as structural changes occur in the muscle itself. Even if the lens changes are the most important, presbyopia is therefore due both to the changes in the lens and to those in the ciliary body.

Epidemiology. Presbyopia affects every person who reaches a more advanced age and is thus the most important age-related phenomenon in the eye overall.

Clinical features. Independent of sex, the ability for near focusing (accommodation distance) of the ocular lens steadily diminishes, practically from early childhood (**Ab**). It usually reaches the "critical limit" of about 4 to 5 D, which is required for comfortable near vision, in middle age (around the age of 45 years). If the ability for near focusing diminishes further, near vision becomes unclear or the near point has to be moved into the distance by moving the observed object (e. g., the newspaper is held farther and farther away, until the required distance exceeds the length of the arm). A certain residual accommodation usually remains until an advanced age. Farsighted (hyperopic) persons usually develop presbyopia sooner than shortsighted (myopic) ones. Presbyopia has no effect on distant visual acuity.

Diagnosis.

The diagnosis is derived primarily from the history. The remaining near vision accommodation can be measured with various devices (e. g., the accommodometer).

Differential diagnosis.

The differential diagnosis occasionally involves **accommodation disorders** from other causes (due to diseases of the ciliary body or lens, diabetes mellitus, or certain medications).

Treatment.

Presbyopia is corrected optically by **near addition** in the form of a converging lens (plus lens, or weakening of any minus correction already present). This usually commences with a near addition of +1 D, which is then increased to + 3 D with increasing age. As the range of sharp vision gets smaller the stronger the glasses, the near addition should be as weak as possible. It is also important to ask about the working or reading distance as the required glasses lens strength depends on this. Separate reading glasses are prescribed for emmetropes. With ametropic, the near addition can be integrated in the distance glasses (bifocal or multifocal lenses). Shortsighted patients sometimes only have to take off their distance glasses to correct their presbyopia. Contact lenses with integrated near addition or surgical procedures on the cornea or with implanted lenses to correct presbyopia have not so far become popular. Medical measures or "eye training" to slow the presbyopia are of no benefit.

A. Presbyopia

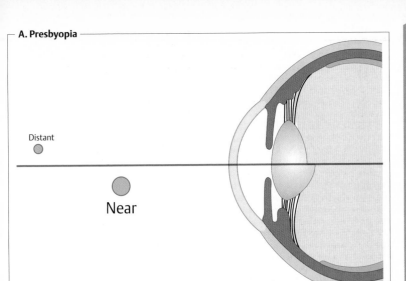

Distant ●

Near

a Upper half of the diagram: eye in condition of disaccommodation (looking into the distance); the ciliary muscle is slack, the zonular fibers are tensed, the lens is flattened (low converging power)
Lower half of the diagram: eye in condition of accommodation (looking at a near object); the contracted ciliary muscle bulges forward in a ring, leading to relaxation of the zonular fibers and thus to increased curvature of the lens because of its intrinsic elasticity (increase in converging power)

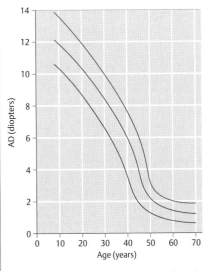

b Reduction in accommodation power (AD) with age (Duane curve)

Presbyopia

137

A. Cataract

Any opacity of the lens beyond the age norm can be called a **cataract**. The term derives from the fact that the ancient Egyptians are said to have believed that the lens opacities were caused by a "membrane" lying over the lens like a waterfall (cataract).

Cataract classification terminology is very varied (see p. 140, **Table 1**). In clinical usage, the different classifications are often combined, e.g., congenital polar cataract, brown nuclear cataract, or mature senile cataract.

Etiology/pathogenesis. The causes of the loss of transparency of the lens are extremely varied (see p. 141, **Table 2**) and largely still not understood. **Photo-oxidative damage** to the lens fiber membranes and the lens proteins is assumed to be the most likely cause of senile cataract – with a protein content of 35 %, the lens is the most protein-rich organ in the human body. In addition there is increasing pigment accumulation in the lens with aging, so that the light absorption maximum shifts to the blue region. High myopia, smoking, heavy alcohol consumption, and high UV light exposure appear to be risk factors for development of senile cataract.

Contusion cataracts are due to contusion-related destruction of lens fibers, while perforations of the capsular sac lead to loss of transparency due to an influx of aqueous humor and swelling of the lens material. The subcapsular, whitish opacities (**"glaukomflecken"**), which occur after acute angle-closure glaucoma, are interpreted as focal pressure-related necrosis of the lens epithelium.

Secondary cataracts (**Ae**) are found predominantly in uveitis, retinitis pigmentosa, intraocular tumors, previous irradiation and corticosteroid therapy. It is suspected that compromise of the equatorial lens epithelium occurs under the influence of the harmful agent, with the consequence that normal lens fiber differentiation ceases and the proliferating lens epithelium migrates in the direction of the (normally epithelium-free) posterior pole, where the cells take on a bubblelike shape (Wedl bubble cells).

Congenital cataracts (**Af**) are an expression of genetic changes, ocular malformations, intrauterine damage (e. g., by infection) or metabolic disorders. In about 25 % of congenital cataracts, family members are affected (usually autosomal-dominant inheritance). The cause of the majority of congenital lens opacities remains unclear.

Epidemiology. Probably more than 90 % of all cataracts are of the senile type (senile cataract). The cataract is therefore a disease mainly of advanced and old age. The transitions between normal age-related loss of transparency of the lens and cataract are fluid, so that figures for the incidence of cataract vary. It can be assumed that about 20–40 % of 60-year-old and 60–80 % of 80-year-old persons have vision-reducing lens opacities, i. e., cataracts. The prevalence of congenital cataract in developed countries is about 2–4 per 10 000 births. All forms of cataract affect both sexes with about the same frequency. The only exception is traumatic lens opacities, which show a marked male predominance. Worldwide, about 20 million persons are blind because of cataract. Cataract is thus the leading cause of blindness. An important task of the world community is to increase the number of cataract operations in the less-developed countries to meet the need.

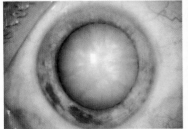

a Mature cataract; the pupil is white

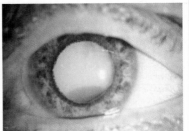

b Hypermature cataract of Morgagni; the brownish nucleus of the lens has sunk downward inside the white liquefied cortical material

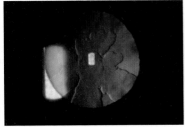

c Intralental water clefts in diabetes mellitus; such lens opacities are sometimes reversible

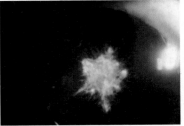

d Syndermatotic cataract: tortoiseshell opacification of the anterior subcapsular parts of the cortex in a patient with atopic dermatitis

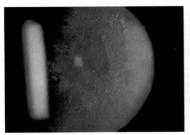

e Opacification of the posterior subcapsular parts of the lens, typically found in secondary cataract

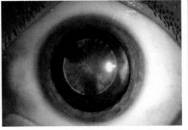

f Opacification of the embryonic lens nucleus in congenital cataract

Cataract

Table 1 Classification (terminology) of lens opacities

- Severity
  - Incipient cataract
  - Advanced cataract
  - Immature cataract
  - Mature cataract (see p. 139, **Aa**)
  - Hypermature cataract with nucleus sunk in the capsular sac (hypermature morgagnian cataract) (see p. 139, **Ab**)
  - Intumescent cataract (with swelling of the lens)

- Location
  - Nuclear cataract (see p. 143, **Ab**)
  - Cortical cataract (anterior or posterior) (see p. 143, **Aa**)
  - Opacities of the outer (subcapsular) parts of the cortex (subcapsular cataract)
  - Opacities of the anterior or posterior pole of the lens (anterior or posterior polar cataract) (see p. 139, **Ad**; see p. 143, **Ac**)
  - Opacities of different layers, (e.g., corticonuclear cataract)

- Shape of the lens opacity, e. g.
  - Wedge-shaped (cuneiform) cataract (see p. 143, **Aa**)
  - Fish-shaped (pisciform) cataract
  - Powdery (pulverulent) cataract
  - Star-shaped (stellate) cataract

- Color
  - Brunescent (brown) cataract (see p. 143, **Ab**)
  - Black cataract

- Time of manifestation
  - Congenital cataract (see p. 139, **Af**; see p. 143, **Ac**)
  - Infantile cataract
  - Juvenile cataract
  - Presenile cataract (in adults under 40 years)
  - Senile cataract (see p. 143, **Aa** and **b**)

- Origin
  - Traumatic cataract
  - Cataract associated with skin diseases (syndermatotic cataract) (see p. 139, **Ad**)
  - Cataract due to other (eye) diseases (secondary cataract) (see p. 139, **Ae**)

Table 2 Causes of lens opacity

- Age (photo-oxidative changes/senile cataract)

- Ocular (mechanical) trauma: blunt (globe contusion) or sharp (penetrating) injury

- Ocular surgery
  - Pars plana vitrectomy
  - Fistulating operations
  - Peripheral iridectomy

- Intraocular diseases
  - Inflammation: chronic uveitis, (infectious) endophthalmitis, rubella embryopathy (Gregg syndrome), syphilis, toxoplasmosis, other
  - Tumors: (anterior) choroidal melanoma, other
  - Degenerative conditions/dystrophies: retinitis pigmentosa
  - Primary intraocular ischemia: following cerclage operation (string syndrome)
  - Acute angle-closure glaucoma ("glaukomflecken")
  - Malformations: microphthalmos, PHPV[a], Peters' anomaly, aniridia, other

- Syndromes
  - Trisomy 13
  - Trisomy 18
  - Trisomy 21
  - Turner syndrome
  - Lowe syndrome
  - Alport syndrome, other

- General diseases
  - Metabolic disorders: diabetes mellitus, galactosemia and galactokinase deficiency, α-galactosidase deficiency (Fabry disease), tetany, myotonic dystrophy (Curschmann-Steinert disease), Refsum syndrome, hepatolenticular degeneration (Wilson disease), defective nutrition, dialysis, other
  - Circulatory disorders: carotid stenosis (ischemic ophthalmopathy), pulseless disease (Takayasu disease)
  - Skin diseases (syndermatotic cataract): atopic dermatitis, Werner syndrome (adult progeria), other
  - Other: neurofibromatosis (NF) type II, premature birth, other

- Medications
  - Corticosteroids
  - Certain cytostatics
  - Chlorpromazine
  - Local parasympathomimetics, other

- Radiation
  - Ionizing: X-rays, β-rays, γ-rays
  - Nonionizing: UV light, infrared rays ("glassblower's cataract"), microwaves, high-voltage current (electric cataract)

[a] PHPV = persistent hyperplastic primary vitreous body

A. Cataract (continued)

Clinical features. The **senile cataract** is usually characterized by wedge-shaped opacities of the lens cortex (cuneiform cataract, **Aa**) and/or initially whitish and subsequently brownish opacities of the lens nucleus ([brunescent] nuclear cataract, **Ab**). Corresponding to the loss of transparency, patients report **cloudy or blurred vision**, reduced contrast, increased glare (scattered light), and changes in color perception (usually a yellowish tinge). Double vision (monocular diplopia) can also occur sometimes because of different refractive indices in the lens. Since it is rather more possible to see past the lens opacities with a dilated pupil, not a few patients complain of more severe symptoms in bright light (sunshine) or when reading, both of which are situations associated with pupil constriction. Overall, cataract-related symptoms are relatively individual and do not correlate absolutely with vision. Some patients already feel markedly disturbed with only slight reductions in lens transparency, while others can still get by well subjectively even with an advanced cataract. Senile cataract is usually bilateral but can be asymmetrical in its severity. Congenital cataracts are bilateral in ca. 65 %.

Typical patterns of opacity are the loss of transparency of the embryonic lens nucleus (nuclear cataract, see p. 139, **Af**), opacities of the anterior or posterior pole of the lens (polar cataract, **Ac**), and opacity of the entire lens (mature cataract). As babies and infants cannot report loss of vision, the gray or white pupil (**leukocoria**) and secondary strabismus are the leading symptoms.

Traumatic lens opacities are usually unilateral. Rosettelike opacities (**contusion or perforation rosette**) are often found. After sharp injuries, defects or (later) scarring of the lens capsule are visible.

Most lens opacities, and particularly the senile forms, usually have a slow progressive course over months and years. Some secondary cataracts may develop relatively quickly. The fastest loss of transparency is found in traumatic openings of the capsular sac (traumatic cataract). Under certain special conditions, lens opacities can regress, e. g., in premature infants (maturing of the lens) or after improvement of the metabolic status in diabetes mellitus or galactosemia. Rarely, an entire opacified lens with the exception of the capsular sac undergoes spontaneous resorption (e. g., after trauma, with rubella cataract, or cataract as part of the Hallermann-Streiff syndrome).

Diagnosis.

The diagnosis is made from the history and slit-lamp appearance, and a mydriatic should be employed to allow assessment of the lens. If the fundus cannot be seen with a very advanced lens opacity, an ultrasound examination of the globe should be performed, at least in the case of unilateral cataract, in order to exclude concomitant ocular diseases such as a tumor or retinal detachment.

Differential diagnosis.

There is no true differential diagnosis. However, very frequently there are additional changes in the eye (e. g., glaucoma, age-related macular degeneration) and it is not always possible to decide how much the cataract contributes to the loss of vision. In the case of congenital cataract, other diseases associated with leukocoria should be considered in the differential diagnosis. The main conditions to be considered are retinoblastoma, Coats disease, Toxocara infection, large choroidal colobomas, persistent hyperplastic primary vitreous body (PHPV), and persistent pupillary membrane (see p. 135, **Ba**).

A. Cataract

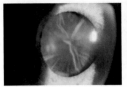

a Cuneiform (cortical) cataract; typical senile cataract

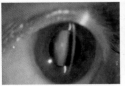

b Brunescent (brown) nuclear cataract; typical senile cataract

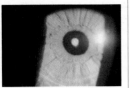

c Anterior polar cataract; these lens opacities are usually congenital

d Scheme of cataract extraction

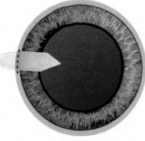

d1 Entering the anterior chamber with a keratome (from temporal side)

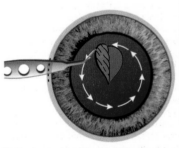

d2 Circular opening of the anterior lens capsule (capsulorhexis)

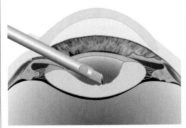

d3 Ultrasonic destruction of the lens nucleus in the capsular sac (phacoemulsification)

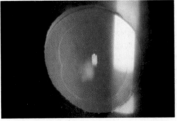

d4 Clinical appearance one day after the operation; the round opening in the anterior lens capsule can be identified with the artificial lens behind it in the capsular sac, the upper edge of which is visible below the pupillary margin

Cataract (continued)

143

A. Cataract (continued)

Treatment. Free-radical scavengers (e. g., vitamin C) are thought to delay cataract development; however, the data in this regard are still very scanty. There are no medications that reverse lens opacities that already are present. As an exception, long-term medical mydriasis may be used (in children) when the paracentral parts of the lens are clear. Treatment of cataract is nearly always surgical.

Cataract extraction is performed when visual acuity has diminished so much that daily life is impaired. From time to time, a lens has to be removed in order to allow better examination and possibly treatment of the ocular fundus (e. g., in diabetic retinopathy). Cataract extraction is usually an elective procedure, but lens-related complications such as **lentogenic (phacomorphic) glaucoma** or inflammation due to lens destruction (**phacolytic uveitis**) can require prompt action. The congenital and infantile acquired cataracts that markedly impair function also require prompt extraction as otherwise underdevelopment of the retina and visual cortex (amblyopia ex anopsia) threatens.

The most popular method of operation today is extracapsular cataract extraction, that is, preserving the capsular sac with ultrasonic destruction of the lens nucleus (**phacoemulsification**) and implantation of an intraocular lens (IOL). The basic sequence of this operation is shown in **Table 1** on p. 145 and is illustrated on p, 143 (**A d1–d4**). When the lens nucleus is very hard, this is slid out from the eye after a larger incision and larger capsule opening by slight pressure (**nucleus expression**). The lens is removed inside the capsular sac (**intracapsular cataract extraction**) only in exceptional cases, usually when the zonular apparatus is insufficient. Since implantation of an artificial lens in or on the capsular sac is then no longer possible, the lack of a lens (**aphakia**) must be corrected by an anterior chamber lens, a lens fixed to the iris, or a posterior chamber lens sutured to the sclera.

Congenital and infantile cataracts can simply be suctioned out as the lens is very soft early in life. The approach is from the front or through the pars plana. Opening the posterior lens capsule (**primary posterior capsulotomy**) and anterior vitrectomy are usually performed in children because of the large risk of secondary cataract and thus risk of amblyopia. Intraocular lenses are inserted with caution in children and usually only after the age of 3 or 4 years when the globe has reached its final length and refraction is thus more stable. Correction of aphakia beforehand is done mostly with contact lenses.

Artificial intraocular lenses are manufactured in varied designs from rigid Plexiglas (polymethylmethacrylate, PMMA) or from soft materials such as acrylates or silicone, which allow the lens to be folded so that it can be inserted through a smaller incision. Most lenses consist of a central optic and usually two footplates (haptics), which serve to center the lens in the capsular sac. Loss of the natural lens is associated with loss of accommodation. Operated patients therefore normally need at least distance or reading glasses. So-called "accommodating" artificial lenses provide only very little accommodation, if any.

"Pseudoaccommodation" can be achieved by multifocal artificial lenses. These lenses are implanted only occasionally and have the disadvantage of somewhat lesser acuity and reduced contrast vision.

In experienced hands, the technical success rate of cataract extraction in otherwise normal eyes is 95–99 %, and the great majority of patients experience a clear gain in function. However, in the usually elderly patient there are frequently concomitant conditions such as macular degeneration, diabetic retinopathy, or glaucomatous optic atrophy, which can limit the improvement in visual acuity. Despite very mature surgical techniques, complications may occur during the operation and also in the short- to long-term postoperative course (p. 146, **Table 2**).

Table 1   Basic course of modern phacoemulsification with intraocular lens implantation

1. Preoperative
   - Explanation of the course without operation, the operation and possible risks.
   - Determine whether the operation will be performed as an ambulatory or inpatient procedure. Concomitant ocular diseases, the patient's general condition, and domestic circumstances should be taken into account.
   - Determine the anesthesia method. The operation is usually performed under local anesthesia (parabulbar anesthesia) or with anesthetic drops (particularly if the patient is on anticoagulant therapy). General anesthesia is necessary in uncooperative patients (e.g., children) or when the initial conditions are very difficult.
   - Echographic measurement of globe length (biometry) and optical measurement of the corneal converging power, followed by calculation of the strength of the artificial lens to be implanted.

2. Intraoperative
   - Administer anesthesia.
   - Exert pressure on the eye (oculopression) to reduce the intraocular pressure and achieve better distribution of the anesthetic (optional).
   - Sterile draping and insertion of a lid speculum.
   - Enter the anterior chamber through the cornea or, after resecting the conjunctiva, through the corneosclera, dissecting a tunnel.
   - Stabilize the anterior chamber by adding a viscous substance (viscoelastic agent).
   - Circular tear of the anterior lens capsule with a curved needle or forceps (capsulorhexis).
   - Injection of liquid between capsule and cortex and between cortex and nucleus (hydrodissection and hydrodelineation).
   - Placement of two stab incisions (paracentesis) to enable bimanual working.
   - Destruction of the lens nucleus in the capsular sac (phacoemulsification).
   - Suction of the soft cortical material with a suction-irrigation system, polishing the capsular sac if necessary.
   - Unfolding of the capsular sac with viscoelastic agent.
   - Implantation of the artificial lens.
   - Suction of the viscoelastic agent.
   - Wound closure by suture provided a self-sealing tunnel was not created.
   - Subconjunctival injection of an antibiotic and corticosteroid for prophylaxis of infection and inflammation.
   - Bandage for a maximum of 1–2 days.

3. Postoperative
   - Ophthalmological examination on first day postoperatively, further examinations as indicated.
   - Inform patient of required behavior (avoidance of direct pressure on the eye).
   - Local therapy until signs of inflammation have subsided.
   - Fitting of new glasses after ca. 2–4 weeks.

Table 2 Complications of cataract surgery

1. Intraoperative
   - Radial tear of the capsulorrhexis or rupture of the posterior lens capsule (incidence ca. 1–3 %). In these cases vitreous prolapse or dislocation of lens material into the vitreous space often occurs, which then necessitates a vitrectomy and makes implantation of an artificial lens difficult.
   - Massive hemorrhage into the choroid or beneath the retina (expulsive hemorrhage) (very rare but often deleterious).
   - Injury to the iris by the phaco handpiece (particularly when the iris is atrophic).
   - Tear of Descemet's membrane.

2. Postoperative
   - Retinal detachment (incidence ca. 1 % with uncomplicated surgery; higher incidence after capsule rupture and with high myopia). Most retinal detachments occur within three years after the cataract extraction.
   - Increase in ocular pressure/glaucoma. In the immediate postoperative period, viscoelastic agent remaining in the eye is the usual cause; this pressure increase is reversible. More prolonged increases in pressure after cataract extraction are rare in adults—lens removal tends to lead rather to a decrease in pressure, but is very common in the long term after lensectomy in childhood (20–40 %).
   - Subacute, acute or hyperacute infection (usually due to bacteria, incidence ca. 1 %) (**Af**).
   - Sterile inflammation with production of fibrin and risk of adhesions (synechiae).
   - Edema of the macula (Irvine–Gass syndrome).
   - Opacity of the cornea (particularly if the endothelial cell density is already reduced preoperatively).
   - Astigmatism (corneal distortion).
   - Wound leakage with reduction in pressure (hypotony) and risk of development of anterior synechia.
   - Trapping of the iris in the wound with irregularity of the pupil.
   - Displacement of the artificial lens, sometimes with iris capture (**Ad** and **e**).
   - Opacity of the artificial lens due to influx of calcium (particularly with soft hydrophilic acrylic lenses) (**Ag**).
   - Intraocular, tumorlike growth of conjunctival or corneal epithelium (very rare).
   - Deterioration of a disease existing before the operation (e. g., diabetic retinopathy, age-related macular degeneration).
   - Opacity of the anterior or, more importantly, the posterior lens capsule due to proliferation of remaining lens epithelium. This secondary cataract occurs in a so-called regeneration variant (with frog's egg-like spheres, **Aa**) and a fibrotic variant (**Ab**) and leads to a late reduction in the initially good visual acuity. The incidence of secondary cataract is between 3 % and 30 % depending on the lens type and operation technique. The treatment of the secondary cataract usually consists of opening the posterior lens capsule by means of a laser (YAG laser capsulotomy, **Ac**). However, retinal detachment is produced in ca. 2% of cases. Surgical procedures can be used sometimes (e. g., suction of secondary cataract).

A. Cataract

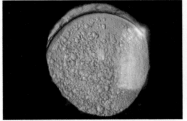

a Secondary cataract of regenerative type (proliferation of the lens epithelium)

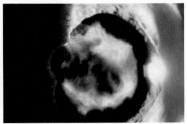

b Secondary cataract of fibrotic type

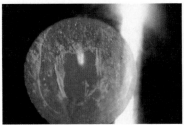

c Appearance after opening the posterior lens capsule (capsulotomy) using a neodymium-YAG laser because of a secondary cataract

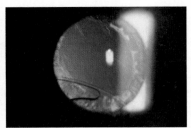

d Considerable downward dislocation of an older artificial lens

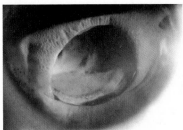

e Anterior displacement of an artificial lens implanted in a child with iris capture

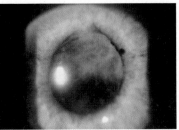

f Infection of the capsular sac after artificial lens implantation

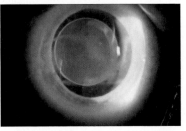

g Opacification of a soft artificial lens (due to influx of calcium)

A. Lens Dislocation

Displacement of the lens within the retro-pupillary plane is called **lens subluxation**. If the lens is loosened so much that it lies in the posterior vitreous space or in the anterior chamber, this is called **luxation of the lens.** The lens displacement overall is also described by the term dislocation.

Etiology/pathogenesis. Subluxation and luxation of the lens are due to partial or total destruction of the zonular apparatus. The cause is mainly trauma and also various metabolic disorders and eye diseases (**A, Table 1**).

Epidemiology. Subluxations and dislocations of the lens are not uncommon and are manifested mainly at a younger age, with the exception of lens displacements due to pseudo-exfoliation (PEX). Traumatic subluxation/ dislocation affects men predominantly, while the metabolically related variants affect the two sexes about equally (A, Table 2). The incidence of lens subluxation/luxation in **Marfan syndrome**, **Weil-Marchesani syndrome**, and **homocystinuria** is ca. 80–90 %.

Clinical features. The patient's symptoms depend particularly on the degree of lens displacement. Slight dislocations often remain asymptomatic. If the lens is displaced so far that the optical axis no longer passes through the lens, then in optical terms the lens is absent (**aphakia**), with a corresponding deficit in converging power. Typical symptoms of lens displacement are **restriction of accommodation**, a reduction in visual acuity, and double vision (diplopia), particularly when the optical axis passes through the periphery of the lens. In many cases, the lens dislocation is associated with a **trembling lens** (**phacodonesis**), visible with the slit lamp.

Diagnosis. The lens displacement can usually be seen readily with the slit lamp (**Aa**). Slight forms of lens dislocation often only become visible when the pupil is dilated. If it cannot be visualized, the position of the lens can be shown by ultrasound.

Differential diagnosis. There is virtually no differential diagnosis. Lens dislocation into the vitreous chamber should be distinguished from surgical or traumatic loss of the lens.

Treatment. The treatment is guided by the symptoms. When the condition is asymptomatic, occasional reexamination is all that is needed. As "repair" of the zonular fibers is not possible, the only possibility to consider when the symptoms are more severe is removal of the lens. As a rule, the capsular sac has to be removed at the same time (intracapsular extraction). The lens can be approached from the anterior chamber or through the pars plana. Correction of the aphakia is preferably by use of an anterior chamber lens or a sclera-fixed posterior chamber lens, sometimes also by contact lenses or cataract glasses. Removal of loosened lenses is associated with an increased postoperative risk of retinal detachment (particularly in Marfan syndrome and high myopia and following trauma). Lenses lying asymptomatically in the vitreous body can be left because they often cause no problems for years or decades. However, complications can arise due to decomposition (phacolysis), so that extraction of such lenses is usually advised in the era of modern vitreoretinal surgical techniques. Lenses dislocated into the anterior chamber (**Ab**) usually cause secondary glaucoma and are therefore an indication for surgery.

A. Lens Dislocation

Table 1 Diseases that can be associated with subluxation or dislocation of the lens

- Sharp and in particular blunt injuries (globe contusion)

- Metabolic disorders
  - Marfan syndrome
  - Homocystinuria
  - Weill–Marchesani syndrome
  - Hyperlysinemia
  - Sulfite oxidase deficiency
  - Ehlers–Danlos syndrome
  - Osteogenesis imperfecta
  - PEX syndrome, others

- Overstretching of the zonular fibers by excessive corneal and/or scleral stretching
  - High myopia
  - Hydrophthalmos
  - Megalocornea
  - Staphyloma

- Other causes/associations
  - Congenital aniridia
  - Mandibulofacial dysplasia
  - Focal dermal hypoplasia
  - Syphilitic uveitis
  - Retinitis pigmentosa
  - Hypermature cataract
  - Intraocular tumors (especially ciliary body melanoma)

- Idiopathic subluxation/dislocation
  - Hereditary
  - Nonhereditary

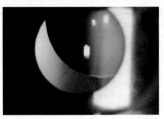

a Subluxation of the lens temporally and upward in a patient with Marfan syndrome; the obviously stretched but still intact zonular fibers can be identified

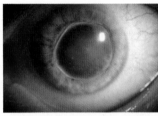

b Dislocation of a completely loosened lens into the anterior chamber

Table 2 Synopsis of the most important syndromes that can be associated with lens dislocation

	Incidence	Manifestation	Direction of the lens subluxation/luxation	Other features to note
Ocular trauma	Very frequent	Any, mainly younger age m >> f	Variable (any direction possible)	Traumatic retinal detachment, traumatic secondary glaucoma
PEX syndrome	Very frequent	Older age m = f	Usually anterior or posterior	PEX glaucoma PEX iridopathy and keratopathy
Idiopathic lens dislocation	Not rare	Usually younger age m = f	Variable	
Lens dislocation in high myopia	Not rare	Usually younger age m = f	Variable	Rhegmatogenous retinal detachment
Marfan syndrome	Not rare	Younger age m = f	Usually temporo-superior, less often naso-superior	Refer to cardiologist (caution: aortic aneurysm), arachnodactyly
Homocystinuria	Rare	Younger age m = f	(Nasal) Downward, often vitreous space	Often spherophakia, tendency for vascular thrombosis
Weill-Marchesani syndrome	Rare	Younger age m = f	Downward, forward	Often small, spherical lens, small stature, brachycephaly

m = male, f = female

A. Inflammation

Inflammation of an intact lens is unknown. Lens protein released by trauma or surgery can provoke **phacogenic uveitis**, where the inflammatory changes (lymphocytes, plasma cells, epitheloid cells, giant cells) are typically most marked in the immediate vicinity of the capsular sac. A lens abscess after (traumatic) introduction of bacteria into the capsular sac is extremely rare.

B. Tumors

The lens is one of the very few tissues in the human body where development of a tumor has never been observed. The lack of malignant transformation capacity of the lens epithelium is probably due to the avascularity of the lens and its position largely isolated from normal metabolism.

C. Trauma

Blunt or sharp injuries of the eye are often responsible for a lens opacity (**traumatic cataract, Ca** and **b**) or lens displacement (see Lens Dislocation, p. 148). About 5% of all intraocular penetrating foreign bodies are in the lens. They are usually removed together with the opacified lens. In certain cases, intralental foreign bodies (with a clear lens center) can be left or extracted with lens preservation. The presence of iron foreign bodies in the lens for a prolonged period may cause rusting of the lens (**siderosis lentis, Cc**). In this case there are typically brownish deposits behind the iris, which only become visible when the pupil is dilated. Copper foreign bodies lead rather to a yellowish-green cataract, which is also called a **sunflower cataract** because of the radially arranged opacities.

D. Spontaneous Lens Resorption and Lens Metaplasia

Under certain conditions a lens can be resorbed spontaneously, especially when it is of a soft consistency. The causes are injuries, inflammation (e.g., rubella embryopathy), certain syndrome-associated forms of cataract (e.g., cataract in **Hallermann-Streiff syndrome**) or **persistent hyperplastic primary vitreous body (PHPV)**. Usually more or less transparent parts of the lens capsule persist.
Fibrous metaplasia of the lens epithelium

sometimes occurs, in which the epithelial cells producing the lens fibers change after inflammation, injury, or surgery into fibrocyte-like contractile cells. In this way, the lens can turn into a tough connective tissue membrane. In PHPV there is replacement of the lens material by fatty tissue in rare cases (pseudophakia lipomatosa, **D**). Ossification of the lens (osseous cataract) is extremely rare. This is usually due to trauma in the distant past that has initiated considerable intraocular transformation processes.

C. Trauma

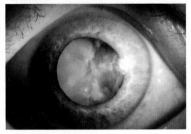

a Opacity and swelling of the lens material after sharp penetrating globe injury

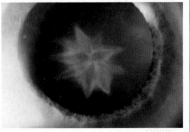

b Rosette-shaped lens opacity after globe contusion (contusion rosette)

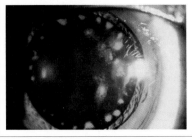

c Circular rust spots beneath the lens capsule (siderosis lentis)

D. Spontaneous Lens Resorption and Lens Metaplasia

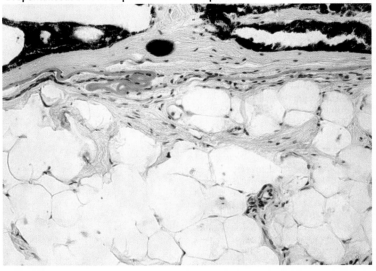

Replacement of the lens by fatty tissue in PHPV with advanced degeneration of the globe; iris remnants at the upper edge of the picture

A. Definition and Classification

For decades glaucoma has been defined primarily as a disorder of aqueous humor dynamics with consequent raised intraocular pressure. More recent discoveries have qualified the significance of the intraocular pressure alone as a pathogenetic factor in the development of glaucoma. According to these, glaucoma must today be defined as an optic neuropathy, which is diagnosed clinically from its characteristic disk appearance and typical changes in the visual field and which can be caused by various risk factors including raised intraocular pressure. It is classified according to etiological and pathogenetic aspects and the classification is usually expanded further by its characteristic course (**A, Table 1**).

B. Diagnosis

Measurement of the **intraocular pressure** is usually performed by applanation tonometry (Goldmann). This measures the force required to flatten the central 7.35 mm^2 of the cornea. The average intraocular pressure is 16.5 mmHg and is subject to a circadian rhythm of ±5 mmHg. Pressures between 25 and 35 mmHg and greater diurnal fluctuations are typical of glaucoma. Thus, a single finding of a pressure of 21 mmHg or less does not exclude glaucoma. Since the thickness of the cornea and other corneal factors has an influence on the intraocular pressure values obtained by applanation tonometry, **measurement of corneal thickness** is being used increasingly for critical scrutiny of the results. The correction factor is 0.2–0.7 mmHg/10 µm (normal 545 µm). Indentation tonometry (Schiötz) and other methods are less used clinically.

Gonioscopy is important in developing the differential diagnosis. Assessment of the chamber angle is made (Spaeth method) according to the width of the chamber angle (10–40°), the shape of the iris curvature (flat, normal, steep) and the level of the iris insertion in the chamber angle (A = high to E = low). In addition, the degree of trabecular pigmentation and anterior synechiae is noted. A range of other classifications is used clinically. Using **ultrasonic biomicroscopy** (UBM), the iris, root of the iris, chamber angle, ciliary body, and lens can also be imaged ultrasonically.

Assessment of the **optic disc** includes noting the size and shape of the disk, the neuroretinal margin and parapapillary, chorioretinal atrophy (zone α and β), and also the depth of cupping, visibility of retinal nerve fibers, diameter of retinal vessels, and the presence of marginal hemorrhages. Glaucomatous optic neuropathy is characterized by the loss of retinal ganglion cells and astrocyte support tissue within the disk, which is shown as an increase in the depth and area of the cupping. Examination is by direct or indirect ophthalmoscopy. Quantification of the loss of neuroretinal tissue is possible by various **morphometric methods**. **Photographic documentation** of the disk and nerve fiber layer facilitates assessment of the disease progress. **Examination of the visual fields** is a crucial part of the investigation. The earliest clinically significant defect is a scotoma, which manifests itself between 10° and 20° from the fixating point (Bjerrum area). As the glaucoma progresses, the scotomas become connected to the blind spot and become confluent. In the late stage, the defects extend to the periphery. Usually the temporal visual field remnant is the last to disappear before the loss of central **visual acuity**. Static threshold perimetry is used particularly for examining the visual field. Kinetic methods are also used for special problems and in advanced disease.

Comprehensive investigation also includes recording the age, medical history (particularly vascular risk factors), and also the family history (see also "Primary open-angle glaucoma," p. 156).

A. Definition and Classification

Table 1 Glaucoma classification proposed by the European Glaucoma Society

- **Primary congenital glaucoma/dysgenetic glaucoma**

- **Primary open-angle glaucoma**
  - Primary open-angle glaucoma with high pressure/chronic simple glaucoma
  - Primary open-angle glaucoma without high pressure/normal-pressure glaucoma
  - Primary juvenile glaucoma
  - Ocular hypertension

- **Secondary open-angle glaucoma**
  - Secondary open-angle glaucoma as a result of ocular diseases
    - Pseudoexfoliation glaucoma
    - Pigment dispersion glaucoma
    - Lens-induced secondary open-angle glaucoma (phacolytic glaucoma, lens particle glaucoma, phacoanaphylactic glaucoma)
    - Glaucoma with intraocular hemorrhage (glaucoma with hyphema, hemolytic glaucoma, ghost cell glaucoma)
    - Glaucoma with intraocular inflammation
    - Glaucoma with intraocular tumors
    - Glaucoma with retinal detachment
    - Traumatic glaucoma
  - Iatrogenic secondary open-angle glaucoma
    - Steroid glaucoma
    - Glaucoma following intraocular surgery and laser therapy
  - Secondary open-angle glaucoma as a result of extraocular diseases
    - Glaucoma with raised episcleral venous pressure

- **Primary angle-closure glaucoma**
  - Primary angle-closure glaucoma

- **Secondary angle-closure glaucoma**
  - Secondary angle-closure glaucoma with pupillary block
  - Secondary angle-closure glaucoma without pupillary block with anterior pulling mechanism
  - Secondary angle-closure glaucoma without pupillary block with posterior pushing mechanism

B. Diagnosis

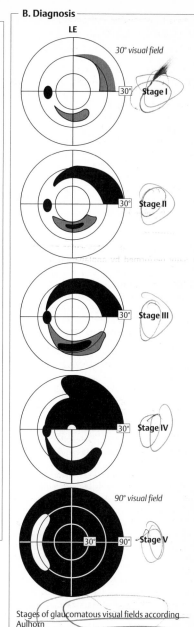

Stages of glaucomatous visual fields according Aulhorn

A. Primary Congenital Glaucoma, Dysgenetic Glaucoma

The dysgenetic or developmental forms of glaucoma are characterized by maldevelopment of the aqueous humor outflow structures, frequently combined with other ocular or systemic conditions.

The cause is disorders of differentiation of the cranial neural tube during the embryonic period. Glaucoma in childhood has an incidence of 1:10 000. The degree of severity and age at manifestation vary greatly. When it is manifested before the age of 3 years it is called congenital glaucoma, and with later manifestation it is called juvenile glaucoma (up to 35 years). The pathologically raised ocular pressure can induce enlargement of the entire eyeball due to the elasticity of the globe that is still present (**buphthalmos**). The diagnostic lead symptom is increased corneal diameter (> 13 mm). Tears of Descemet's membrane and subsequent repair mechanisms lead to typical corneal scars (**Haab bars**). Other symptoms are epiphora and photophobia. It is classified according to syndromatological or morphological aspects.

In about 50 % of glaucomas in childhood and youth, there is isolated **trabecular dysgenesis**, in which there is an obstruction to aqueous humor outflow without further ocular and systemic anomalies (**Aa**). Three chamber angle formations are distinguished: posterior, anterior, and concave iris insertion. Schlemm's canal is usually patent. The morphological and functional severity is highly variable. Spontaneous remissions in the form of secondary maturation of the chamber angle have been described.

Iridotrabecular dysgenesis is explained by the common origin in an association of cells in the cranial neural tube. Dysgenetic findings in the iris can be represented by iris stromal hypoplasia, persistent pupillary membrane, iris hyperplasia (including ectropion uveae), or pathological iris vessels (irregular, superficial iris vessels, persistence of the vascular tunic of the lens), as holes, as iris colobomas or as aniridia (**Ab–d**).

Peripheral, midperipheral, and central forms of **iridocorneotrabecular dysgenesis** (**Ae** and **f**) can be distinguished; posterior embryotoxon is the name of the prominent margin of Descemet's membrane, which is found as a fine whitish ring in the peripheral cornea in 15–30 % of normal eyes. If peripheral, mesodermal strands from the iris stroma to Schwalbe's line also occur; this is called **Axenfeld's anomaly**. In 50 % of cases, glaucoma occurs due to displacement of the chamber angle (Axenfeld syndrome). In **Rieger's anomaly**, midperipheral anterior synechiae and iris stromal hypoplasia are characteristic in addition to posterior embryotoxon. Pupillary ectopia, corneal opacities, and glaucoma (50 % of cases) can also occur. Additional dental or skeletal anomalies characterize Rieger syndrome. As the transition between Axenfeld's and Rieger's anomalies is fluid and the two conditions often occur together, it is assumed that they are variants of the same malformation complex, collectively termed the Axenfeld-Rieger syndrome. The central form of iridocorneotrabecular dysgenesis is called **Peters' anomaly**. This is a rare and usually bilateral anomaly. Dysgenetic glaucoma occurs in 50–70 % of eyes. There are also central corneal opacities, absence or thinning of individual corneal layers, anterior synechiae of iris and lens, anterior polar cataract, and microphthalmos. Additional malformations of the CNS, heart, circulation, or facial skeleton are called Peters-plus syndrome.

Typical **systemic malformations**, in which development of dysgenetic glaucoma occurs, are Lowe syndrome, phakomatoses (especially Sturge-Weber syndrome), Rubinstein-Taybi syndrome, Pierre-Robin syndrome, chromosome aberrations, Marfan syndrome, Weil-Marchesani syndrome, rubella embryopathy, and homocystinuria.

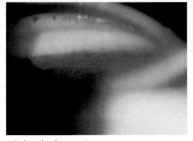

a Trabecular dysgenesis

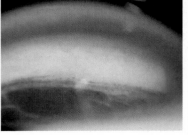

b Iridotrabecular dysgenesis

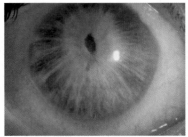

c Iridotrabecular dysgenesis

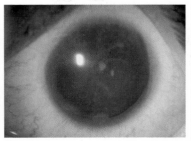

d Aniridia

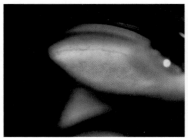

e Iridocorneotrabecular dysgenesis

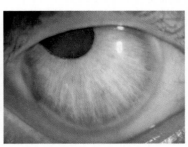

f Iridocorneotrabecular dysgenesis

A. Primary Open-Angle Glaucoma

Simple chronic glaucoma (primary open-angle glaucoma with high pressure, primary chronic open-angle glaucoma) is characterized by an intraocular pressure greater than 21 mmHg (**Aa**), an open chamber angle (**Ab**), characteristic disk cupping (**Ac–e**) with visual field defects (**Af**), and the absence of a known secondary cause of glaucoma. The rise in the intraocular pressure is caused by an increased resistance to outflow in the juxtacanalicular trabecular meshwork. Associated gene mutations (MYOC/TIGR) have been found increasingly in recent years. Primary chronic open-angle glaucoma is the most common form of glaucoma. The prevalence is about 1.4% in the population over 40 years of age. There is no sex predisposition. Twenty percent of all cases of blindness in the Western world are caused by simple glaucoma. The disease begins insidiously and has no symptoms initially until already obvious visual field defects have occurred. In most cases suspicion is aroused by a routinely detected abnormal appearance of the disk. Without treatment, the intraocular pressure is usually between 25 and 35 mmHg. The chamber angle is widely open. The disease is chronic and slowly progressive. Untreated it leads to gradual loss of ocular function.

B. Normal-Pressure Glaucoma

The important feature of normal-pressure glaucoma is the presence of glaucomatous optic neuropathy and visual field defects with intraocular pressure in the normal range, an open chamber angle, and the absence of a known secondary cause of glaucoma. The term includes an entire group of glaucomas. Numerous risk factors (compression of the optic nerve, vascular dysregulation, arterial hypertension and hypotension, sleep apnea syndrome, and alterations in blood rheology, viscosity, and coagulability) can influence its development and/or course. Furthermore, genetic associations (optineurin) are increasingly coming to light, which allow a better distinction from primary chronic open-angle glaucoma. The prevalence in Western Europe is about 0.6%. The diagnosis is made mainly as a diagnosis of exclusion of other forms of glaucoma and nonglaucomatous optic neuropathies. Nevertheless, the intraocular pressure plays a part in the pathogenetic events. A reduction in the pressure by 30% or more can prevent or at least slow further progression of the disease. Progression of the glaucomatous damage despite effective pressure lowering should suggest a major nocturnal drop in blood pressure. If there is persistent evidence that a vasospastic syndrome is present, systemic therapy with magnesium in mild cases and with low-dose calcium-channel blockers in more severe forms can be given. Cooperation with the primary care doctor is advisable in any case.

C. Primary Juvenile Glaucoma

Primary juvenile glaucoma occurs between the ages of 10 and 35 years. While it follows a similar clinical course, it shows a greater genetic dependence than primary chronic open-angle glaucoma. Associated genes have been found on chromosome 1 and MYOC. There is often a positive family history.

D. Ocular Hypertension

Ocular hypertension is characterized by intraocular pressure levels greater than 21 mmHg without characteristic glaucomatous optic neuropathy. Measurement of corneal thickness is required for critical evaluation of pressures measured by applanation tonometry. Only a minority of persons develop glaucomatous damage in the course of years. The five-year conversion rate is about 10%. Treatment is advisable if there are additional risk factors.

A. Primary Open-Angle Glaucoma

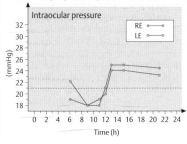

a Pressure profile in primary open-angle glaucoma

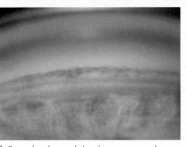

b Open chamber angle in primary open-angle glaucoma

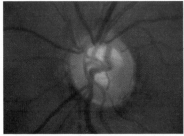

c Advanced optic neuropathy in primary open-angle glaucoma

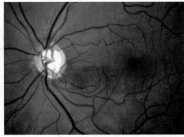

d Defects in the nerve fiber layer in primary open-angle glaucoma

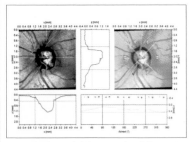

e Scanning laser ophthalmoscopy (Heidelberg retina tomography) in primary open-angle glaucoma

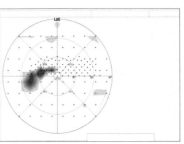

f Visual field defects in primary open-angle glaucoma

A. Secondary Open-Angle Glaucoma

Secondary open-angle glaucoma is characterized by increased intraocular pressure with progressive, typically glaucomatous optic neuropathy and visual field defects; it occurs as a consequence of an ocular or extraocular disease and/or treatment. The chamber angle is open more than 270°. Transition to secondary angle-closure glaucoma is frequent.

Pseudoexfoliative syndrome is characterized by deposition of pseudoexfoliation material in the anterior segment of the eye and in various extraocular tissues. About 20–60% of the patients develop glaucoma (pseudoexfoliative glaucoma (**PEX glaucoma**) through obstruction of the trabecular meshwork. The pseudoexfoliation material is a fibrillary basement membrane protein, for the origin of which genetic and nongenetic causes (UV radiation, autoimmune factors, slow virus infection, trauma) are believed responsible. Patients in the 5th to 6th decades are mainly affected. There is an increased prevalence in persons of Scandinavian ancestry. An increased familial incidence has been described. PEX glaucoma usually manifests itself with markedly higher pressure levels, more rapid progression, and lower pressure tolerance than in primary chronic open-angle glaucoma. The PEX material appears as gray-white flakes and is found on the corneal endothelium, the iris, lens, zonular fibers, and ciliary body processes as well as in the intratrabecular and intertrabecular spaces of the trabecular meshwork (**Aa, b**). Occasionally, phacodonesis or spontaneous dislocation of the lens can be seen. Gonioscopically, increased pigmentation of the chamber angle can be seen and sometimes there is a wavy line anterior to Schwalbe's line (Sampaolesi line). Glaucomatous optic neuropathy is also found corresponding with increased intraocular pressure levels. As in primary chronic open-angle glaucoma, this is a chronic progressive disease, but it shows a reduced response to conservative therapy, so it usually leads to early surgical intervention.

Pigment dispersion syndrome is characterized by pigment deposition in the anterior segment of the eye. Through overloading of the trabecular meshwork, with a subsequent alteration in the trabecular lamellae, about 25–35% of patients develop glaucoma (**pigment dispersion glaucoma**). According to the theory of inverse pupillary block, the iris acts as a valve, causing the intraocular pressure in the anterior chamber to be higher than in the posterior chamber. This leads to the peripheral iris being pressed back against the lens. Release of melanin granules occurs because of friction between zonular fibers and the back of the iris. Myopic men aged 30–40 years are predominantly affected. Pigment glaucoma usually develops within the first 15 years after the pigment dispersion is found. In some cases there is a rise in intraocular pressure on physical exertion or after pupil dilatation, presumably as a result of increased pigment dispersion. Typically, spindle-shaped to triangular pigmentation of the corneal endothelium with its base inferior is seen (**Krukenberg spindle, Ac**). The trabecular meshwork is highly pigmented (**Ad**). Because of the loss of pigment from the iris pigment epithelium, radial transillumination defects occur (**church window phenomenon, Ae**). Dustlike pigment deposits can also be apparent on the anterior surface of the iris, lens, zonular fibers, and retinal periphery. If a rise in intraocular pressure also occurs, characteristic glaucomatous optic neuropathy can develop. Ultrasonic biomicroscopy is helpful in diagnosing inverse pupillary block (**Af**). Like primary chronic open-angle glaucoma, this is a chronic progressive disease. Besides local pressure-lowering therapy, laser iridotomy or surgical iridectomy to abolish the inverse pupillary block is recommended. Spontaneous remissions are possible.

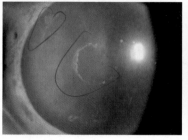

a Pseudoexfoliative glaucoma

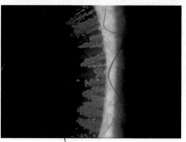

b Pseudoexfoliative glaucoma

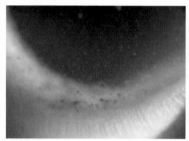

c Krukenberg spindles in pigment dispersion glaucoma

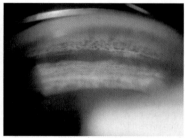

d Appearance of chamber angle in pigment dispersion glaucoma

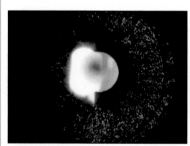

e Church window phenomenon (transillumination defects) in pigment dispersion glaucoma

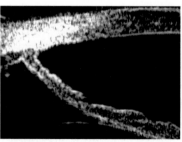

f Ultrasonographic biomicroscopic appearance in pigment dispersion glaucoma

A. Secondary Open-Angle Glaucoma (continued)

Phacolytic glaucoma is occasionally observed with mature or hypermature cataract (**Aa**). Denatured lens protein passes through the intact lens capsule and is phagocytosed. Obstruction of the trabecular meshwork by macrophages or lens protein leads to an increase in outflow resistance with a subsequent rise in intraocular pressure. **In lens particle glaucoma** the obstruction of the trabecular meshwork is due to lens particles from a lens injured by trauma or surgery. **Phacoanaphylactic glaucoma** is characterized by granulomatous inflammation of the trabecular meshwork after complication-free extracapsular cataract extraction because of an existing sensitization to released lens protein.

Anterior chamber hemorrhage (**hyphema**) leads to an increase in intraocular pressure through obstruction of the trabecular meshwork (**Ab**). **Hemolytic glaucoma** arises from obstruction of the trabecular meshwork by macrophages, which phagocytose the erythrocyte degradation products. After vitreous hemorrhages, the erythrocytes degenerate into so-called **ghost cells**, which enter the anterior chamber through defects in the anterior vitreous limiting membrane, where, and because of the loss of their natural deformability, they can displace the trabecular meshwork and increase outflow resistance.

During the acute phase of anterior or intermediate **uveitis**, the intraocular pressure can fall to subnormal levels as the inflammation of the secretory ciliary epithelium leads to a reduction in aqueous humor production. In the further course, however, inflammation-induced glaucoma frequently develops due to an increase in the viscosity of the aqueous humor as a result of increased protein content, obstruction of the trabecular meshwork by inflammatory cells, or swelling of the trabecular meshwork cells in the course of trabeculitis. The increased outflow resistance leads to an increase in intraocular pressure. With chronic inflammation (**Ac**), neovascularization, adhesions, and scarring can occur. Secondary angle-closure glaucoma develops as a result of anterior synechiae. Important forms that are associated with an increase in intraocular pressure are Fuchs heterochromic cyclitis and Posner-

Schlossman syndrome, and also uveitis in juvenile idiopathic arthritis, herpes simplex, herpes zoster, or Behçet disease.

Glaucoma with intraocular tumors arises because of tumor extension into the trabecular meshwork and/or obstruction of the trabecular meshwork by tumor-related neovascularization, inflammation, necrosis, hemorrhage, or pigment dispersion (**Ad**). The clinical features and course are very variable.

Although **retinal detachment** is usually associated with a drop in intraocular pressure, secondary reorganization processes can also cause a rise in intraocular pressure.

The **traumatic forms of glaucoma** are a heterogeneous group of glaucoma diseases, in which not only the type of ocular trauma is important but numerous different pathogenetic processes are also involved. Treatment is difficult and the results are often unsatisfactory. Sometimes, glaucoma develops only years later. Transient rises in intraocular pressure occasionally occur following **intraocular surgery** and **laser treatment** due to persistence of viscoelastic substances, lens particles, vitreous prolapse, or prostaglandin secretion. With the increasing use of silicone oil in vitreoretinal surgery, the number of cases of silicone oil glaucoma due to displacement of the trabecular meshwork is increasing (**Ae**).

Glaucoma with raised episcleral venous pressure (**Af**) arises as a result of intravascular outflow obstruction or because of arteriovenous shunts. In contrast to other forms of glaucoma, the cause of the increase in outflow obstruction is distal to Schlemm's canal.

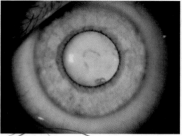

a Phacolytic glaucoma with mature cataract

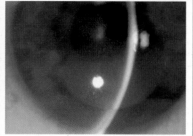

b Glaucoma with hyphema and hematocornea

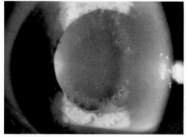

c Glaucoma with chronic uveitis

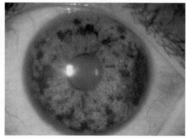

d Glaucoma with malignant melanoma of the iris

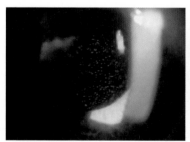

e Silicone oil glaucoma with emulsified silicone oil bubbles in the anterior chamber

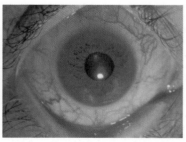

f Glaucoma with raised episcleral venous pressure

A. Primary Angle-Closure Glaucoma

Primary angle-closure glaucoma is a collective term for closure of the chamber angle by a range of different mechanisms in the absence of a known secondary cause of the rise in intraocular pressure. The shift in aqueous humor outflow leads to structural changes in the eye as well as a rise in intraocular pressure. Acute angle closure is characterized by reversible iridocorneal apposition; in contrast, chronic angle closure arises on the basis of irreversible anterior synechiae.

The most common pathological mechanism is pupillary block (**Aa**); the shift in the transpupillary aqueous humor outflow produces a rise in pressure in the posterior chamber. Because of this, the peripheral iris is pressed against the trabecular meshwork and Schwalbe's line. The circular obstruction of the trabecular outflow causes a rise in intraocular pressure to levels up to 80 mmHg. Anatomical (lens size, corneal diameter, axis length) and physiological (pupil size) factors are predisposing. In the rare plateau iris mechanism (**Ab**) when there is a very thick and/or flat peripheral iris and with anterior iris insertion, the iris root can obstruct the trabecular aqueous humor outflow in mydriasis. The central anterior chamber depth is often not reduced. The diagnosis is made by ultrasonic biomicroscopy. Iridotomy and iridectomy are often ineffective for plateau iris. Improvement can be achieved by giving strong miotics. Further systemic risk factors for pupillary block include female sex, a positive family history, and sympathomimetic and sympatholytic therapy.

Acute angle-closure glaucoma (glaucoma attack, **Ac**) is the result of a reversible, sudden and complete closure of the chamber angle, usually as a consequence of a pupillary block mechanism. The patients complain of rapidly progressive deterioration in vision and pain and redness of the affected eye. Nausea, vomiting, and cardiac arrhythmias can also occur. Morphologically there is mixed injection with corneal edema, a shallow anterior chamber, and positive Tyndall effect; the medium-sized to dilated pupil is often oval in shape and does not react to light and the disk is hyperemic. The attack can be interrupted by miotics, carbonic anhydrase inhibitors, and hyperosmotics. Causal treatment (both eyes) is given in the at-

tack-free interval by means of laser iridotomy or surgical iridectomy (**Ad, e**). In most cases, the intraocular pressure can be reduced to normal levels by this means permanently and without medication. If more than 50 % of the chamber angle is closed, further therapy with local antiglaucoma agents is occasionally necessary. The cumulative risk of a glaucoma attack in the other eye is 10 % per year.

Intermittent angle-closure glaucoma describes a form of angle-closure glaucoma in which the symptoms of acute angle closure are milder but occur recurrently.

Chronic angle-closure glaucoma is characterized by irreversible, slowly progressive obstruction of the chamber angle. Obstruction of the trabecular outflow usually begins above and spreads downward gradually. The intraocular pressure is usually only moderately raised, and disk changes and visual field findings resemble those of primary chronic open-angle glaucoma.

As a consequence of the mechanical damage during the acute rise in pressure, foci of iris atrophy and pupil irregularity are found after acute angle closure. The chamber angle can be open or closed to a varying degree. Small, gray-white subcapsular lens opacities (**glaukomflecken, Af**) are evidence of previous acute angle closure. The pressure damage can lead to pale optic atrophy. Untreated or treated too late, angle-closure glaucoma leads to permanent impairment of ocular function or even painful blindness.

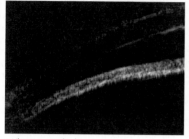

a Ultrasonographic biomicroscopic appearance with narrow anterior chamber

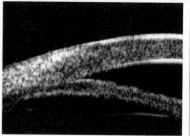

b Ultrasonographic biomicroscopic appearance with plateau iris

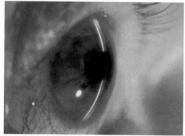

c Acute angle closure

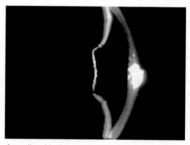

d Pupillary block before laser iridotomy

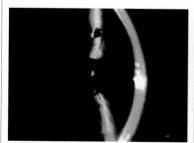

e Pupillary block after laser iridotomy

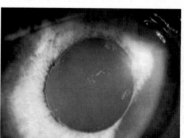

f Glaukomflecken

A. Secondary Angle-Closure Glaucoma

Secondary angle-closure glaucoma is further classified according to its pathomechanism. Pupillary block signifies obstruction of trabecular outflow by the peripheral iris due to displacement of the transpupillary aqueous humor outflow with a consequent rise in the pressure in the posterior chamber of the eye. Secondary angle-closure glaucoma with pupillary block occurs with lens swelling, anterior lens dislocation, posterior synechiae, vitreous protrusion in aphakia (**Aa**), microspherophakia, and intraocular lenses (**Ab**). Secondary angle-closure glaucoma with anterior ("pulling") mechanism is found after trauma, surgical procedures, and inflammation, as well as neovascularization glaucoma and ICE (iridocorneal endothelial) syndrome. The trabecular meshwork is displaced by iris tissue or a membrane, which gradually narrows the chamber angle by contraction and finally closes it.

Neovascularization glaucoma (**Ac**) is a typical complication of retinal hypoxia, such as that which occurs in proliferative diabetic retinopathy, central retinal vein or central retinal artery occlusion, Eales disease, untreated retinal detachment, severe intraocular inflammation, or tumors, leading to the formation of new vessels. The neovascularization proliferation commences typically at the pupillary margin and continues from there radially toward the chamber angle (**rubeosis iridis**) until the new vessels join up with the circulus arteriosus iridis major. From there, proliferation extends over the surface of the ciliary body and the scleral spur deep into the trabecular meshwork (**Ad**). Peripheral anterior synechiae occur early through contraction of the newly formed fibrovascular tissue. The ocular pressure begins to rise. Through progressive contraction of the fibrovascular tissue there is gradually complete obstruction of the chamber angle. The iris is pulled over the entire trabecular meshwork. Pupil distortion and ectropion uveae are the result. The intraocular pressure rises further and markedly. Pain develops along with congestive hyperemia of the entire globe. Neovascularization glaucoma is characterized by a sometimes fulminant course. Along with the obligatory treatment of the underlying disease, early surgical intervention is often necessary. The prognosis is poor. Enucleation is regarded as a last resort.

Iridocorneal endothelial (ICE) syndrome (**Ae**) is the collective term for essential (or progressive) iris atrophy, iris nevus (or Cogan-Reese) syndrome, and Chandler syndrome, which are different manifestations of the same disease. Starting from a primary corneal endothelial change, a membrane consisting of endothelial cells and Descemet-like cells grows out over the open chamber angle and onto the anterior surface of the iris. Contraction of the membrane leads to the development of anterior synechiae, pulling the pupil toward the synechiae, and to iris atrophy and the development of iris holes in the opposite quadrant. Glaucoma develops because of obstruction of the chamber angle (**Af**). The loss of regular endothelial cells leads secondarily to corneal decompensation with painful restriction of vision. A viral etiology is suspected. Middle-aged women are affected predominantly. The disease is unilateral and there is no increased familial incidence. Therapeutically, along with conservative and surgical treatment of the glaucoma, penetrating keratoplasty is the primary treatment when there is severe reduction in vision.

Secondary angle-closure glaucoma due to posterior ("pushing") mechanisms occurs because of forward displacement of the iris-lens diaphragm and the associated narrowing of the trabecular meshwork. Posterior mechanisms are found in malignant glaucoma, iris and ciliary body cysts, intraocular tumors, silicone oil or gas in the vitreous cavity, uveal effusion, retinopathy of prematurity, and various congenital anomalies.

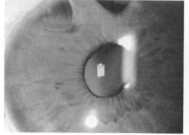

a Aphakia glaucoma

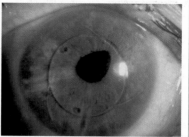

b Glaucoma with anterior chamber lens

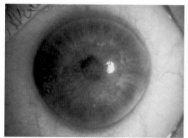

c Neovascularization glaucoma

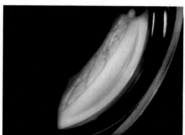

d Appearance of chamber angle in neovascularization glaucoma (secondary angle-closure glaucoma)

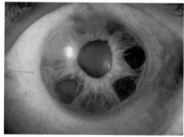

e ICE syndrome

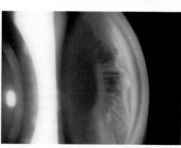

f Appearance of chamber angle in ICE syndrome

A. Drug Treatment

The goal of glaucoma treatment is avoidance of further progression of the disease by lowering the intraocular pressure by at least 30% and to levels below 18 mmHg. The first-line therapy is usually drug treatment. Various types of drugs are currently in use, some of which are available as combined preparations. All locally applied antiglaucoma drops share local intolerance reactions and local cytotoxic effects. **Sympathomimetics** (nonselective/α-selective) lower the intraocular pressure by reducing the production of aqueous humor and improving outflow. **Sympatholytics** (β-selective) lower the intraocular pressure by reducing aqueous humor production. The effect commences after two hours and lasts about 24 hours. Systemic side-effects include in particular cardiac arrhythmias and bronchospasm, which is why preexisting arrhythmias and chronic obstructive lung diseases are contraindications. **Carbonic anhydrase inhibitors** also lower the intraocular pressure by reducing the production of aqueous humor. The effect commences after only an hour and lasts up to 12 hours. A typical systemic side-effect with oral administration is hypokalemia due to diuretic loss of potassium. With systemic therapy, potassium should therefore be replaced. **Parasympathomimetics** (cholinergics) lower the intraocular pressure by reducing outflow resistance. In addition, they have a pupil-constricting effect. **Prostaglandin derivatives** lower the intraocular pressure by improving the uveoscleral outflow path. Typical local side-effects are dark coloration of the eyelashes and iris, increased growth of the lashes, and conjunctival hyperemia. **Osmotic agents** are the most effective reducers of intraocular pressure. They are given intravenously in acute angle closure.

B. Surgical Treatment

A surgical procedure is indicated when the medical reduction in pressure is inadequate or progression occurs despite apparently well-controlled ocular pressure. In **neodymium-YAG laser iridotomy** a small hole is created in the iris without opening the eye as in surgical **iridectomy**. By this means an equalization of pressure between the posterior and anterior chamber can be created in acute angle closure; the anterior chamber becomes deeper and outflow through the trabecular meshwork is again possible. **Argon laser trabeculoplasty** creates a cicatricial contraction in the vicinity of the trabecular meshwork, thus widening the outflow passages. The effect is usually temporary, similar to **cyclophotocoagulation**, in which atrophy of parts of the aqueous-producing ciliary body is achieved using a laser. The effect usually commences within the first few weeks. The treatment can also be carried out with heat (cyclodiathermy), high-frequency ultrasound, or cold (cyclocryocoagulation). By the creation of a corneoscleral tunnel, the aqueous humor is diverted under the conjunctiva in **trabeculectomy**, where a filtering bleb develops (**Ba**). The success rate has been markedly improved by use of antimetabolites (mitomycin, 5-fluorouracil) that influence postoperative wound healing. There is a range of variations of this most common surgery of glaucoma therapy. In contrast, **deep sclerectomy** and **viscocanalostomy** are not perforating, penetrating operations since parts of Schlemm's canal and the trabecular meshwork remain intact. **Cyclodialysis**, **goniocurettage**, and **trabecular aspiration** have not so far become accepted clinically. The status of **drainage implants** (**Bb**) and **retinectomy** in the most severe and treatment-refractory forms of glaucoma has not yet been finally clarified. In congenital glaucoma, **goniotomy** or **trabeculotomy** is performed.

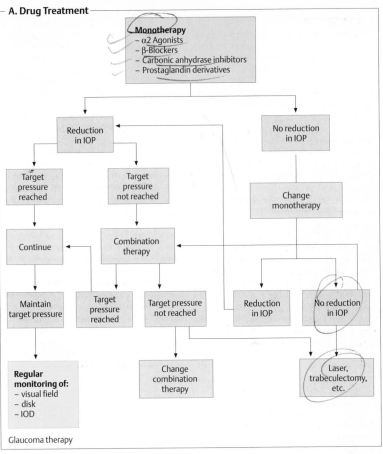

A. Drug Treatment

Monotherapy
- α2 Agonists
- β-Blockers
- Carbonic anhydrase inhibitors
- Prostaglandin derivatives

Reduction in IOP

No reduction in IOP

Target pressure reached

Target pressure not reached

Change monotherapy

Continue

Combination therapy

Maintain target pressure

Target pressure reached

Target pressure not reached

Reduction in IOP

No reduction in IOP

Regular monitoring of:
- visual field
- disk
- IOD

Change combination therapy

Laser, trabeculectomy, etc.

Glaucoma therapy

B. Surgical Treatment

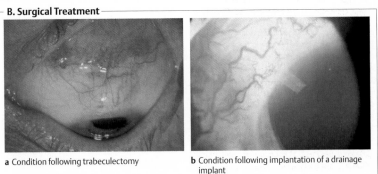

a Condition following trabeculectomy

b Condition following implantation of a drainage implant

A. Coloboma

A retinochoroidal coloboma is characterized by a cleft directed downward. The cause of this congenital anomaly is incomplete closure of the fetal optic cup cleft. Colobomas are bilateral in over 60% of patients. A well-demarcated, oval, yellow-white lesion is visible usually in the lower temporal half of the fundus (**A**). It can extend as far as the disk and macula. The iris or lens can be involved. Microphthalmos, high myopia, cataract, and phthisis bulbi can be associated. The visual prognosis depends on the extent of the coloboma and the presence of other anomalies. Amblyopia, nystagmus, and strabismus are common. Secondary choroidal neovascularization and retinal detachment are complications of chorioretinal coloboma.

B. Myelinated Nerve Fibers

Myelinated nerve fibers are congenital intraretinal nerve fibers containing myelin; 80% of cases are unilateral. A juxtapapillary bright white feathered lesion is often apparent (**B**). They are located in the inner layers of the retina, and usually occur as isolated lesions at the posterior pole or mid-periphery. Papilledema, papillitis, retinal inflammation, and cotton wool spots should be excluded in the differential diagnosis. Central visual acuity is rarely affected.

C. Capillary Hemangioma of the Retina (von Hippel Disease, Retinal Angiomatosis)

A retinal capillary hemangioma can present at the periphery of the retina or at the edge of the disk. The tumor is a reddish or whitish, prominent, round lesion with feeder vessels (**C**). Hard exudates, exudative detachment, fibrovascular proliferation, and hemorrhages can be visible depending on whether there is leakage from the tumor. If other organs (cerebellum, kidney, adrenal, pancreas) are affected, it represents hereditary von Hippel-Lindau disease. A general examination of the patient and family screening are therefore essential. Treatment consists of laser photocoagulation, cryotherapy, photodynamic therapy, brachytherapy, and vitrectomy.

D. Retinoblastoma

Retinoblastoma is the most common malignant ocular tumor in childhood. It originates from primitive retinoblasts. The gene responsible for retinoblastoma is located on chromosome 13q14. The incidence is 1:14 000 live births. The average age at diagnosis is 18 months and 67% of cases are unilateral. The most common presentation of retinoblastoma is leukokoria (50%), strabismus (20%), reduced vision, red eye, glaucoma, and an orbital cellulitis-like picture. The retinoblastoma grows endophytically (subretinally) (**Da**) or exophytically (into the vitreous space (**Db**). On ultrasound a solid mass with high internal echoes is seen. The classification in the tumor tissues can be shown ultrasonographically and by CT, and the differential diagnosis of other causes of leukokoria is important (see below). On histopathology, rosettes (Flexner-Wintersteiner, **Dc**, and Homer-Wright) and fleurettes confirm the diagnosis. The therapy options are laser photocoagulation, thermotherapy, cryotherapy, external radiotherapy, brachytherapy, chemotherapy, and enucleation. The affected families require detailed genetic counseling. The prognosis of retinoblastoma depends on invasion of the optic nerve and choroid. The mortality is ca. 8% in the absence of optic nerve invasion; this rate increases to 45% when tumor invasion extends to behind the lamina cribrosa.

E. Leukokoria

Leukokoria is the name for a white reflex seen in the pupillary aperture. Leukokoria requires precise differential diagnosis. Possible causes are primary hyperplastic persistent vitreous body, Coats disease, ocular toxoplasmosis, retinoblastoma, retinal detachment, cataract, and endophthalmitis.

A. Coloboma

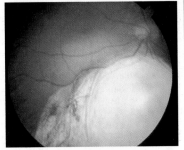

Retinochoroidal coloboma in the lower half of the fundus

B. Myelinated Nerve Fibers

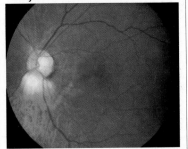

Myelinated nerve fibers below the disk

C. Capillary Hemangioma

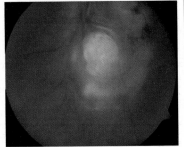

Capillary hemangioma of the retina with feeder vessels

D. Retinoblastoma

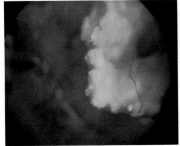

a Calcified retinoma (possibly regressed retinoblastoma)

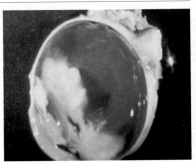

b Exophytic retinoblastoma (macroscopic appearance following enucleation)

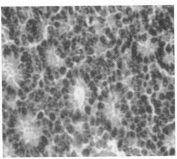

c Flexner–Wintersteiner rosettes in retinoblastoma

A. Degenerative Conditions and Age-related Changes

Vitreous liquefaction. With increasing age, liquefaction of the gel-like vitreous body takes place. This begins in front of the macula or in the center of the vitreous. It is found in over 90% of those over 40 years. Earlier occurrence is observed with myopia, uveitis, trauma, and surgery, and in some hereditary syndromes.

Posterior vitreous detachment. Following vitreous liquefaction, the posterior vitreous body limiting membrane becomes detached from the retina (Aa). The membrane is attached at the disk by a ring-shaped structure, which is visible in the vitreous space as a mobile ring (Weiss ring) following detachment. This is regarded as certain evidence of vitreous detachment. Patients often perceive this structure as a transparent mobile object in front of the eye. A posterior vitreous detachment is apparent in 25% of 60- to 69-year-olds. This rate increases to over 60% between 70 and 79 years. Premature vitreous detachment can also develop with high myopia and following cataract surgery, intraocular inflammation, and trauma.

Vitreous hemorrhage. Following an acute posterior vitreous detachment, separation of the vitreous gel often occurs at the base of the vitreous in the upper quadrants of the retina. If the pull of the vitreous leads to bleeding into the vitreous space, a mirror-image hemorrhage is often seen in the lower periphery at the margin of the vitreous where it is still attached (Ab).

Equatorial degeneration (palisades). Equatorial degeneration is seen in ca. 4.5% of emmetropic and ca. 17% of myopic eyes over 6 diopters. These lesions can appear circular, in the region of the posterior equator, or else radial along a peripheral retinal vessel. Multiple atrophic round holes often become visible in the palisade. Nevertheless, so-called horseshoe holes, which occur at the edge of the palisade, are the usual cause clinically of rhegmatogenous retinal detachment.

White with pressure/white without pressure. These terms refer to a well-demarcated whitish lesion in the retinal periphery. If it can be demonstrated by the examiner only by depressing the retina, it is called "white with pressure." If it is visible without additional manipulation, it is called "white without pressure." There is no increased risk of retinal detachment. Nevertheless, prophylactic laser treatment is recommended if the other eye has previously developed a giant tear of the retina.

Pavingstone degeneration. This is the term for well-demarcated areas of pigment epithelium atrophy located in the retinal periphery. There is no association with the development of a primary retinal tear.

Retinoschisis. In retinoschisis there is a split in the neurosensory retina. Typical retinoschisis (splitting in the external plexiform layer) commences in the ora serrata as cystoid degeneration (Ac). In the reticular type of retinoschisis, splitting occurs in the innermost layers of the neurosensory retina. Retinoschisis is commonly bilateral and located in the lower quadrants of the retinal periphery. The incidence is 4–10%. Holes are seen in the external layers in over 20% of eyes with retinoschisis. In contrast, holes in the internal layers are very rare. Retinoschisis is often benign and does not require any treatment. The risk of progressive schisis detachment is 1%. In contrast to retinal detachment, retinoschisis shows a transparent, rigid surface and does not move with ocular movements, and there are white spots within the schisis cavity on laser application. Progressive schisis detachment is treated by buckle surgery or pars plana vitrectomy.

Asteroid hyalosis. In this condition there are numerous yellowish round particles in the vitreous, which move together with ocular movements (Ad). It is unilateral in 70% and of no pathological significance. Vision is not impaired.

Synchysis scintillans. This involves numerous small yellow structures in the vitreous space. The condition is often bilateral. After eye movements, the particles sink; they have no negative effect on visual acuity.

A. Degenerative Conditions and Age-related Changes

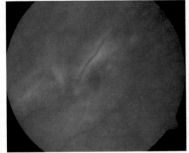

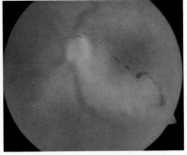

a Vitreous detachment with avulsed retinal vessels and retinal break; laser spots visible around the break

b Vitreous hemorrhage with posterior vitreous detachment

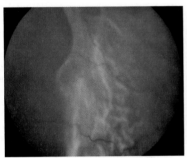

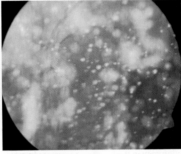

c Retinoschisis with breaks in the outer layer

d Asteroid hyalosis

A. Retinal Detachment

Retinal detachment is the term for detachment of the neurosensory retina from the retinal pigment epithelium through influx of fluid into the subretinal space. Different forms (rhegmatogenous, exudative, tractional) are distinguished.

B. Rhegmatogenous Retinal Detachment

Rhegmatogenous (= break-induced) retinal detachment is produced by a full-thickness defect (hole). It is an ophthalmological emergency, which can lead to blindness if untreated.

Etiology/pathogenesis. The most common causes are age-related destruction and liquefaction of the vitreous body. The vitreous detachment following degeneration can cause holes and tears through traction (vitreous pull) on the peripheral retina, through which the liquid part of the vitreous can penetrate and separate the neurosensory layer from the pigment epithelial layer. Other predisposing factors are high myopia, cataract surgery, and ocular trauma.

Epidemiology. The incidence of rhegmatogenous retinal detachment is 0.01%. It is diagnosed most frequently between the ages of 50 and 70 years. The risk of rhegmatogenous retinal detachment in the opposite eye is 10%.

Clinical features. The most important symptoms are photopsia (flashes in the eye), floaters ("mouches volantes"), and an absolute scotoma ("shadow"). If the macula is not affected (**Ba**), visual acuity can be relatively good. Clinically, the detached retina shows a whitish and creased surface (**Ba–c**). Retinal defects, pigment cells, and erythrocytes are found in the vitreous body often with subnormal intraocular pressure.

Diagnosis. The diagnosis is made clinically by indirect ophthalmoscopy with mydriasis. The goal of the examination is to detect all causative retinal breaks. If no retinal break is seen, ultrasonography is necessary to exclude possible exudative retinal detachment. Types of retinal tears:

- *Horseshoe tear* (**Bd**). The anterior part of the retina is elevated by vitreous traction. A bridging vessel may be seen. The risk of retinal detachment is high.
- *Round hole with operculum.* The operculum lies free above the retinal hole. There is no vitreous pull at the edges of the hole, so the risk of detachment is low.
- *Atrophic hole.* Often a round retinal hole is seen in the middle of a palisade without vitreous pull. The risk of retinal detachment is low.
- *Dialysis.* The retinal defect is seen in the region of the ora serrata. The cause is often trauma (see "Retinal detachment with dialysis of the ora," p. 174).

C. Exudative Retinal Detachment

In exudative retinal detachment, the separation of the neurosensory retina from the pigment epithelium is the result of increased leakage of fluid from intraocular tumors, of a disturbance of the blood-retina barrier, or of mechanical block of the venous outflow of the retina.

Etiology/pathogenesis. Choroidal or retinal tumors (hemangioma, malignant melanoma, retinoblastoma, retinal angiomatosis, metastases, peripheral vasoproliferative retinal tumors); systemic diseases (leukemia, advanced arterial hypertension, renal failure, preeclampsia); vascular retinal diseases (ischemic central vein occlusion, Coats disease, choroid ischemia); inflammation (scleritis, Harada disease, orbital Echinococcus). A systemic screening should be performed to exclude distant metastases if a tumor is suspected.

Diagnosis. The boundaries of the exudative detachment change with position (in contrast to rhegmatogenous and tractional detachment) and the surface is smooth. It is often seen in the lower half of the fundus (**C**). A prominent mass, strikingly dilated retinal veins, or other signs of inflammation are symptoms indicative of exudative detachment.

B. Rhegmatogenous Retinal Detachment

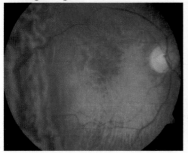

a Retinal detachment in the temporal mid-periphery without macular involvement

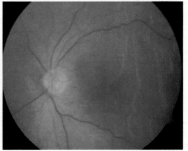

b Subtotal retinal detachment with macular involvement

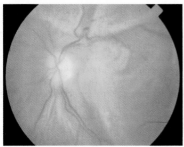

c Total retinal detachment

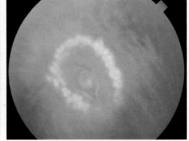

d Horseshoe-like break with bridging vessel surrounded by laser spots

C. Exudative Retinal Detachment

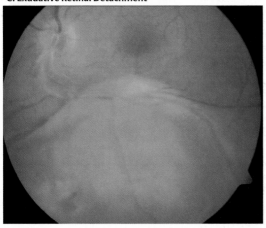

Inferior exudative retinal detachment with retinal vascular abnormality

A. Tractional Retinal Detachment

In tractional retinal detachment, the detached retina shows a rigid, concave surface. After-movements of the retina are absent. Epiretinal membranes and star folds of the retina are additional characteristic findings.

The most common causes are **proliferative vitreoretinopathy** (diabetes mellitus, vascular occlusions of the retina, detachment operation, trauma), persistent vitreous traction, and hereditary vitreoretinal diseases.

B. Special Forms of Retinal Detachment

Retinal detachment with dialysis of the ora. In 85 % of retinal detachments after blunt ocular trauma, there is a tear of the ora serrata. Interruption of the insertion of the retina in the ora serrata develops. Eighty percent of the detachments are diagnosed within two years after the trauma. The superonasal or inferotemporal quadrants are affected most frequently. Progression of the ora dialysis is insidious because of the firm consistency of the vitreous body in young patients. The treatment of choice is buckling parallel to the limbus combined with cryosurgery (see below).

Giant tear detachment. A circular tear of the retina over more than 90° of the circumference is called a giant tear. It is mostly idiopathic or develops after blunt or surgical ocular trauma. Other causes are vitreoretinal dystrophy (Wagner-Stickler disease) and acute retinal necrosis. Men are affected more often. The disease is often bilateral. Various procedures (buckle surgery with or without intraocular gas injection, pars plana vitrectomy with silicone oil endotamponade) are possible. The other eye must be monitored regularly. Prophylactic treatment of abnormal peripheral areas of the retina in the other eye is recommended, particularly in the presence of high myopia and vitreous traction.

Retinopathy of prematurity (retrolental fibroplasia, ROP). This is a vasoproliferative vitreoretinopathy, which in those affected can lead to detachment even in childhood and youth. ROP affects preterm infants who are exposed to high oxygen concentrations. This can interrupt the normal vascular development of the immature retina. As a result, undesirable vasoproliferative processes occur (active ROP), which turn into a scarring stage with vitreous and epiretinal traction.

Preterm infants with a birth weight of less than 1500 g or with a gestational age of less than 32 weeks are at high risk of developing ROP. Retinal detachments in the first month of life are usually tractional or exudative. Rhegmatogenous detachment develops only after a few years, with changes in the gel-like vitreous body.

The stages of ROP have been defined in an international classification (**Table 1, Ba–c**). Although the majority of affected children show spontaneous regression, progression of the ROP can lead to blindness. The treatment depends on the stage, severity, and location of the pathological changes. Therapeutic options include cryotherapy, laser coagulation, buckle surgery, and vitrectomy.

Proliferative vitreoretinopathy (PVR). PVR develops following migration and proliferation of pigment cells, glial cells, macrophages, and fibroblasts in the vitreous body and on the retinal surface (epiretinal and subretinal). The resulting membrane structures lead to tractional retinal detachment (**Bd**). It is frequent with long-standing retinal detachments and after failed surgery for detachment. Other risk factors are the number, size, and location of the retinal tears, previous laser coagulation or cryotherapy of the retinal tears, and repeated intraocular surgery. Depending on the severity of the PVR, a denting procedure can produce anatomical success in ca. 40 % of the patients. A success rate of over 75 % can be achieved by combination with vitrectomy. The functional results are very modest even after retinal attachment is achieved.

B. Special Forms of Retinal Detachment

Table 1 Stages of retinopathy of prematurity

Stage	Clinical features
I	Demarcation line (between the healthy and avascular retina)
II	Ridged demarcation line
III	Ridged demarcation line with extraretinal fibrovascular proliferation
IV a b	Incomplete retinal detachment – Without macula involvement – With macula involvement
V	Total tractional retinal detachment; may be funnel-shaped

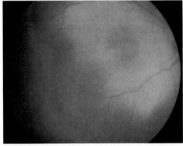

a Demarcation line with extraretinal neovascularization in ROP, stage III

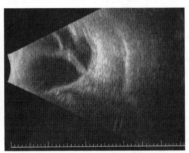

b Ultrasonic funnel-shaped retinal detachment in ROP, stage V

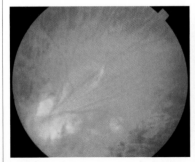

c Retinal detachment in spontaneously regressing ROP

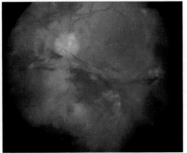

d Tractional retinal detachment in PVR

A. Treatment of Rhegmatogenous and Tractional Retinal Detachment

The general aims of treatment are induction of an adhesion around the retinal tear, restoration of contact between the detached neurosensory retina and the retinal pigment epithelium, and elimination of tractional forces.

Various methods are employed depending on the location of the hole, the age of the patient and of the detachment, the appearance of the fundus, and the surgeon's experience. Rhegmatogenous retinal detachment is an emergency. Following the diagnosis, the patient should remain fasting so that surgery can be performed as soon as possible. A ban on reading until the operation and placing the patient on the side of the hole (e. g., flat and on the right with a horseshoe tear at the 10-o'clock position in the right eye) is recommended as this can counteract further progression of the detachment until the time of surgery.

B. Scleral Buckling Procedure

After marking the retinal defect on the outer sclera, cryosurgery is performed around the lesion. This is followed by approximation of the globe wall to the detached retina through a depression of the globe wall by fixing a segmental buckle or a circular band (cerclage over 360°) to the sclera. The advantages of buckle surgery are the basic technical equipment, the short rehabilitation time, the low risk of iatrogenically induced lens opacity, and avoidance of intraocular complications such as hemorrhage or inflammation (particularly when no aspiration is performed to drain the subretinal fluid). The limitations are a reduced view of the fundus (e. g., with miosis), multiple retinal holes in different quadrants and limbus distances, large and central retinal tears, and scleral thinning.

C. Pneumatic Retinopexy

In pneumatic retinopexy (**C, Table 1**) an inert expanding gas or air is injected into the vitreous. In this way, the retina is reattached. Cryosurgery is performed before or after the gas injection or laser coagulation is done around the retinal defect after attachment of the retina. Detachments with a single retinal tear in the upper periphery of the fundus (10-o'clock to 2-o'clock positions) are the best precondition for this procedure.

D. Pars Plana Vitrectomy (PPV)

Under the operating microscope, the vitreous body and all epiretinal and subretinal tractional components are removed. The retina is then reattached by application of liquid perfluorocarbon. The retinal defects are sealed with endolaser or exocryoapplication. The perfluorocarbon is then exchanged for silicone oil or expanding gases to tamponade the retina. A second operation is required to remove the silicone oil.

Advantages of PPV are the precise location of all retinal holes, elimination of media opacities, the fact that it can be combined with cataract extraction, direct relief of vitreous traction, and removal of epiretinal and subretinal strands.

Disadvantages of PPV are the expensive equipment and experienced team needed, slow opacification of the lens (cataract), the possibility of a second operation to remove the silicone oil, and the necessity for early postoperative follow-up (fibrin reaction in the anterior chamber, increased intraocular pressure).

Expanded indications for PPV. Primary procedure in rhegmatogenous pseudophakia and PVR detachment; macular diseases (macular hole, choroidal neovascularization, macular edema); to obtain material in inflammatory and infiltrative diseases; endophthalmitis; retinal vascular occlusion (e. g., arteriovenous decompression in branch vein occlusion); tumor endoresection; therapy-refractory glaucoma; internal reconstruction after globe trauma.

C. Pneumatic Retinopexy

Table 1 Characteristics of expanding gases used within the eye

Gas	Expansion	Intraocular use	Intraocular duration
SF_6, sulfur hexafluoride	2	20 %	10 – 14 days
C_2F_6, perfluoroethane	3,5	16 %	30 – 35 days
C_3F_8, perfluoropropane	4	16 %	55 – 65 days

D. Pars Plana Vitrectomy

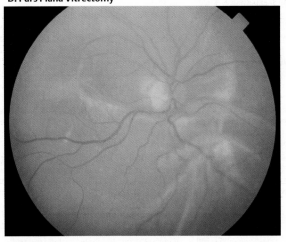

PVR ablation with subretinal disturbance

Table 2   Classification of proliferative vitreoretinopathy

Grade	Location	Characteristics		
A	Vitreous body	Opacities and pigment cell clumps in the vitreous body (mainly inferior)		
B	Retinal surface	Wrinkling of the inner retinal surface, rolled retinal hole edges, increase in vessel tortuosity; rigid retina; decrease in vitreous body motility		
C	Posterior	1 – Focal	Stellate fold
		2 – Diffuse	Confluent stellate folds; optic nerve often not visible
	Posterior or anterior	3 – Subretinal	Subretinal proliferation; "napkin ring" strands around the optic nerve; dendritic "washing lines," "motheaten" plaques
	Anterior	4 – Circular	Contraction along the posterior edge of the base of the vitreous body; retina pulled in the direction of the vitreous body; posterior radial folds in the retina
	Anterior	5 – Anterior displacement	Vitreous body pulled forward; stretching of the ciliary body; iris retraction; hypotony

A. Central Retinal Vein Occlusion (CRVO)

CRVO is the second most common vascular disease of the retina after diabetic retinopathy. Retinal hemorrhages, dilatation, and increased tortuosity of the retinal veins are seen in all four quadrants.

Etiology/pathogenesis. Arterial hypertension is the most important predisposing systemic disease; diabetes mellitus, cardiovascular diseases, hyperviscosity syndromes, and increased intraocular pressure are other risk factors. On histopathology, thrombosis is seen within the central retinal vein at the level of the lamina cribrosa.

Epidemiology. There is an increased incidence of CRVO between the fifth and seventh decades.

Clinical features. The perfusion of the retina determines the clinical features of the CRVO (see below).

Nonischemic CRVO (venous stasis retinopathy, nonhemorrhagic CRVO, perfused CRVO, **Aa** and **b**). The capillary nonperfused area of the retina is smaller than 10 disk areas. The reduction in vision is caused by the edema or hemorrhages in the macula. When the central visual acuity on first presentation is 0.5 or better, the visual prognosis is good in over 67 % of patients. Nevertheless, up to 34 % of nonischemic CRVO can convert within 32 months to ischemic CRVO.

Ischemic CRVO (hemorrhagic CRVO, nonperfused CRVO, **Ac**). The capillary nonperfused area is greater than 10 disk areas. Extended retinal hemorrhages and cottonwool spots are found at the disk margin and at the posterior pole. Marked disk swelling is common in the acute stage. The causes of reduced vision are edema, hemorrhage, and ischemia in the macula, neovascular glaucoma, vitreous hemorrhage, and exudative or tractional retinal detachment. Two major complications of ischemic CRVO are rubeosis iridis and neovascular glaucoma.

Diagnosis. The clinical appearance is often sufficient for diagnosis. Fluorescence angiography demonstrates the area of retinal ischemia to be measured so that classification of the CRVO is possible. Afferent pupillary defects and electroretinography are additional diagnostic methods for assessing the retinal ischemia in the acute stage of CRVO.

Treatment. *Observation:* In the case of nonischemic CRVO without macular edema, there should be monthly follow-up to allow early diagnosis of the occurrence or increase of retinal ischemia. Besides ophthalmoscopy, slit-lamp examination of the anterior segment and tonometry are essential to promptly identify the most feared complications (rubeosis iridis, chamber angle neovascularization, neovascular glaucoma).

Medical: Regulation of high blood pressure and the treatment of risk factors have a beneficial effect on the prognosis. The acceptance of platelet aggregation inhibitors, isovolemic hemodilution, and systemic corticosteroids varies.

Laser photocoagulation: Panretinal laser photocoagulation is recommended according to the "Central Retinal Vein Occlusion Study Group" in the presence of the following findings:

- Retinal ischemia over 10 disk areas
- Neovascularization of the retina
- Neovascularization of the iris greater than two clock hours
- Chamber angle neovascularization

Surgical: Radial optic neurotomy, intravitreal steroid injection. These new surgical procedures have not yet been evaluated by prospective randomized studies.

B. Branch Retinal Vein Occlusion (BRVO)

Hemorrhages and edema of the retina are found in the region of the affected retinal veins (**Ba**). The occluded retinal vein is dilated peripheral to the site of arteriovenous crossing. Reduced vision and sectoral visual field defects result from hemorrhages, edema, or retinal ischemia (**Bb, c**). If there is a perfused macula with edema, grid laser photocoagulation is indicated. Sectoral laser coagulation is recommended in retinal neovascularization, ischemia over five disk areas, or rubeosis iridis.

A. Central Retinal Vein Occlusion (CRVO)

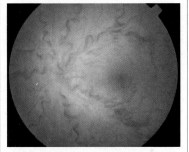

a Venous stasis retinopathy (nonischemic CRVO)

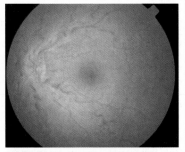

b Venous stasis retinopathy after 12 months with regression of the hemorrhages and edema

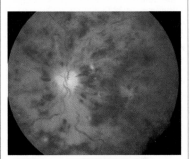

c Ischemic CRVO (hemorrhagic CRVO) with marked hemorrhages and edema

B. Branch Retinal Vein Occlusion (BRVO)

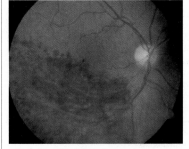

a Occlusion of the inferior temporal vein

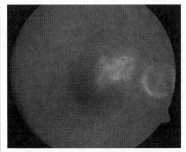

b Fluorescence angiography shows perfused macular edema (acute stage) with occlusion of the superior temporal vein

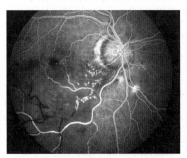

c Fluorescence angiography shows retinal ischemia below the macula with occlusion of the inferior temporal vein

A. Central Retinal Artery Occlusion (CRAO)

CRAO is caused by occlusion of the central artery of the retina. The lead symptom is painless and sudden reduction in vision.

Etiology/pathogenesis. There is usually an embolus or thrombus. A yellow cholesterol embolus (Hollenhorst plaque) on the head of the optic nerve or in a branch retinal artery confirms the diagnosis. The most important causes of emboli are atherosclerotic plaques of the carotid arteries, arterial hypertension, and cardiac valve lesions.

Epidemiology. The prevalence of CRAO is 0.85 per 100 000 population in one year. It is a disease of adulthood (in the sixth decade of life on average). Involvement is bilateral in 1–2%, with the exception of temporal arteritis and other systemic vasculitides.

Clinical features. Visible emboli in the retinal arteries and cherry-red reflection (dark red foveal appearance surrounded by whitish retinal edema at the posterior pole, **Aa**, **b**) is pathognomonic of central retinal artery occlusion. The arteries are thin and the segmented blood flow in the retinal arteries can be observed in acute stages of the disease (**Ac**).

Diagnosis. Diagnosis is made clinically (see below). The diagnosis can be confirmed by fluorescence angiography.

Differential diagnosis. Differentiation between arteritic (Horton disease) and nonarteritic CRAO is very important because in Horton disease the fellow eye can become involved within a few days without appropriate treatment.

Treatment. There is no consensus currently about the efficacy of different forms of treatment.

- *Conservative treatment:* globe massage, anterior chamber paracentesis, infusion treatment with pentoxifylline, hyperbaric oxygen, intravenous rTPA, or corticosteroid injection.
- *Invasive treatment:* selective catheterization of the ophthalmic artery with administration of fibrinolytic drugs.

Prognosis. The visual acuity on first presentation generally decides the prognosis. Spontaneous improvements are observed in up to 15%.

B. Branch Retinal Artery Occlusion (BRAO)

Corresponding to the occluded arterial branch, retinal edema is more apparent at the posterior pole (**Ba**). Patients report a sector-shaped visual field defect. The reduction in central visual acuity depends on the perfusion of the fovea (**Bb**). Besides the whitish retinal edema, yellowish intra-arterial emboli and narrowing of the arteries are important clinical findings. Screening for cardiovascular risk factors and conservative therapy (see CRVO, p. 178) are recommended. The prognosis for central visual acuity is good.; however, visual field defects can persist.

C. Ocular Ischemic Syndrome

This is chronic insufficiency of the ophthalmic artery leading to reduced perfusion of the entire eye. The most common cause is **carotid stenosis**. Central visual acuity is reduced in the advanced stages. Clinically, narrowed retinal arteries and dot-and-blot hemorrhages in the periphery of the retina are apparent. Dilatation and tortuosity of the retinal veins are absent (differential diagnosis: venous stasis retinopathy). Rubeosis iridis and a Tyndall effect in the anterior chamber are common. The retinal neovascularization often develops following rubeosis iridis. The pathologically prolonged arm-retina filling time on fluorescence angiography is pathognomonic. Carotid Doppler examination can show the extent of the stenosis. Affected patients usually show a high-risk profile with regard to cardiovascular diseases. The mortality is ca. 50% within five years after the diagnosis is made. Evaluation by an internist is therefore strongly recommended. Panretinal laser photocoagulation is performed in the case of extensive retinal ischemia and in the presence of rubeosis iridis and retinal neovascularization.

A. Central Retinal Artery Occlusion (CRAO)

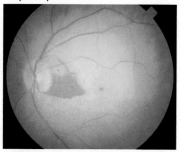

a CRAO with retinal edema due to ischemia; intact retinal perfusion temporal to the disk is due to the patent cilioretinal artery

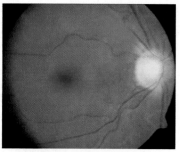

b CRAO with cherry-red spot in the fovea

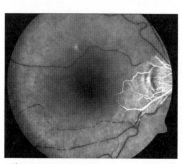

c Fluorescence angiography with nonperfused area of the retina and segmented blood flow

B. Branch Retinal Artery Occlusion (BRAO)

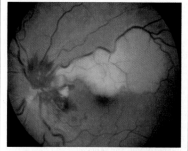

a BRAO with retinal edema corresponding to the sector supplied by the superior temporal artery; retinal hemorrhage at the edge of the disk, dilatation and tortuosity of the veins indicates combined arteriovenous occlusion of the retina

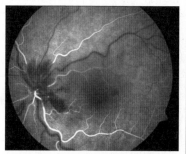

b Fluorescence angiography shows the nonperfusion of the retina

A. Arterial Macroaneurysm of the Retina

Round dilatations of the retinal arterioles within the first three orders of arteriolar bifurcation are called acquired arterial macroaneurysms. Arterial hypertension and atherosclerosis are the most important causes. The condition is usually unilateral and is more frequent in women. A reduction in vision or a visual field defect occurs when there is leakage or hemorrhage in the region of the macula. Hemorrhages can occur in different layers of the retina and in the vitreous space. Subpigment epithelial hemorrhages show as dark red lesions and require differential diagnosis from pigmented choroid tumors. If multiple macroaneurysms, inflammatory cells in the vitreous, or collateral vessels are found, a precise diagnosis is important because the prognosis and the treatment of the arterial macroaneurysms can vary (see Coats disease below; branch retinal vein occlusion, p. 178). Arterial macroaneurysms can often be shown by indocyanine green angiography despite epiretinal hemorrhages. The hemorrhages are nearly always reversible. If there is a reduction in vision following resorption of the hemorrhages, fluorescence angiography is recommended to show leakage from the macroaneurysm. Laser photocoagulation of the macroaneurysm can then lead to resolution of the leakage.

B. Coats Disease

Coats disease is a congenital retinal vascular disease characterized by retinal telangiectases, microaneurysms, and capillary hypoperfusion areas in the periphery of the retina. Miliary aneurysms of the liver and certain forms of idiopathic juxtafoveal telangiectases are regarded as variants of Coats disease. Histopathologically there is a loss of endothelial cells and pericytes of the retinal vessel walls. Male are affected predominantly. Eighty percent of cases are unilateral. There is an increased incidence of the disease in the first and fifth decades of life. Peripheral retinal vascular anomalies cause leakage, which presents at the posterior pole in the advanced stage as macular edema and subretinal lipid deposits (**Ba, b**). Coats disease is a chronic, slowly progressive disease. The diagnosis is usually made by the exudation at the posterior pole. Complications are retinal detachment, vasoproliferative tumor of the retina, cataract, glaucoma, and phthisis bulbi.

The diagnosis is made clinically and by the demographic features (sex, age) and the fluorescence angiographic appearance in the retinal periphery (**Bc**). The differential diagnosis includes other causes of leukokoria in childhood and peripheral retinal vasculopathies in adults. The treatment of Coats disease is based on destruction of the avascular areas of the retina and leaking microaneurysms. The treatment of choice is laser photocoagulation. Cryotherapy is employed if laser therapy fails, if the lesions are located at the extreme periphery of the retina, or if there is an increase in the subretinal exudations. In the advanced stage of Coats disease (exudative retinal detachment, vasoproliferative tumor formation), vitreoretinal procedures are also possible.

C. Hypertensive Retinopathy

Chronic arterial hypertension leads to narrowing of retinal arterioles and a disturbance of the internal blood-retina barrier. As a result, exudates, hemorrhages, cottonwool spots, and lipid deposits develop with a preference for the posterior pole of the retina. The stages of hypertensive retinopathy (according to Scheie) are:

Stage 0: Normal retinal appearance.

Stage I: Diffuse arteriolar narrowing. No focal change in the caliber of the arterioles.

Stage II: Marked arteriolar narrowing with additional focal constrictions (**Ca**).

Stage III: Marked diffuse and focal arteriolar narrowing with retinal hemorrhages.

Stage IV: In addition to the listed findings, retinal edema, hard exudates, and papilledema occur (**Cb**).

A. Arterial macroaneurysm of the Retina

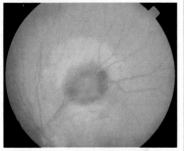

Arterial macroaneurysm in the course of the superior temporal artery; retinal, subretinal, and subretinal pigment epithelial hemorrhages can be seen

B. Coats Disease

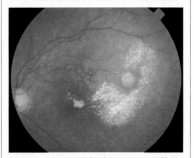

a Macular edema with lipid deposits caused by arterial microaneurysms

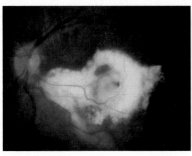

b Submacular cholesterol plaque in Coats disease

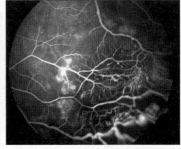

c Fluorescence angiography in Coats disease: retinal telangiectases, microaneurysms, capillary breakages with leakage at the periphery

C. Hypertensive Retinopathy

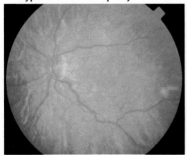

a Stage II hypertensive retinopathy

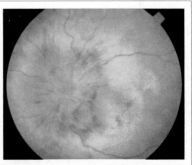

b Stage IV hypertensive retinopathy with papilledema and macular star

A. Diabetic Retinopathy

Diabetic retinopathy (DR) is a microangiopathy of the retina caused by insulin deficiency.

Etiology/pathogenesis. The following metabolic disorders are produced in diabetes mellitus by hyperglycemia: sorbitol cycle, nonenzymatic glycation and production of AGEs (advanced glycation end products), activation of DAG/PKC (diacyl glycerol/protein kinase C).

Diabetic retinopathy is characterized by microvasculopathy. Microvascular changes seen are: thickening of the basement membrane, loss of pericytes, and reduction in extracellular matrix. As a result of these changes, microaneurysms, retinal edema, retinal ischemia, and retinal neovascularization can develop.

The cytokine VEGF (vascular endothelial growth factor) is an important factor in the pathogenesis of diabetic retinopathy. The occlusion of retinal capillary vessels and the resulting hypoxia lead to increased release of VEGF. VEGF then induces retinal neovascularization and leakage from retinal vessels.

Epidemiology. In developed Western countries, the rate of blindness in diabetic retinopathy is ca. 8 % in individuals under 65 years old. It is almost twice as high (14.5 %) among 65- to 74-year-old patients.

Diagnosis. Funduscopic examination with mydriasis is crucial.

Stage classification of DR.

Nonproliferative DR (NPDR, **Aa** and **b**):

- *Mild form:* isolated microaneurysms
- *Moderate form:* retinal hemorrhages and/or microaneurysms at the posterior pole and/or hard exudates
- *Severe form:* in addition to the mild or moderate forms, retinal hemorrhages and microaneurysms in four quadrants, venous beading in two quadrants, or intraretinal microvascular abnormality (IRMA) in one quadrant

Proliferative DR (PDR):

- *Neovascularization of the disk* (NVD): new vessels on or within one disk diameter of the disk
- *Neovascularization elsewhere* (NVE); **Ac–e**): New retinal vessels more than one disk diameter distant from the disk

Clinically significant macular edema. Retinal thickening within 500 µm of the center of the macula, or lipid deposits within 500 µm of the center of the macula associated with a thickening of the adjacent retina; thickening of the retina over at least one disk area size and located within one disk diameter from the center of the macula. **4:2:1 rule.** Numerous microaneurysms in all four quadrants or venous beading in at least two quadrants or IRMA in at least one quadrant. The changes indicate severe diabetic retinopathy.

Treatment.

Laser therapy: The concept of laser photocoagulation (LC) in PDR is based on downregulation of VEGF production by ablative therapy of ischemic areas of the retina. By converting the hypoxia to anoxia, regression of retinal neovascularization can be achieved. Focal laser photocoagulation is employed in nonischemic forms of diabetic macular edema. The indications are:

- NPDR (severe form): panretinal LC
- PDR: panretinal LC
- Clinically significant macular edema: focal LC

Through prompt and effective laser therapy, the risk of severe loss of vision can be prevented in up to 60 %. In clinical routine, focal laser photocoagulation of clinically significant macular edema is performed before the panretinal laser photocoagulation (see p. 187, **Tables 1 and 2**, **Aa–c**).

The complications of panretinal laser photocoagulation are visual field defects, nyctalopia, disorders of contrast and light sensitivity, and an increase in macular edema.

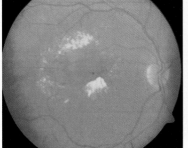

a Clinically significant macular edema at the posterior pole in NPDR

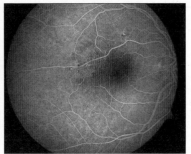

b Fluorescence angiography shows numerous microaneurysms in the macula

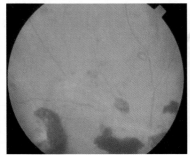

c Venous looping and NVE with preretinal hemorrhage

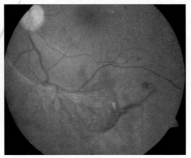

d NVE with glial proliferation

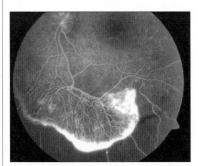

e Fluorescence angiography shows leakage at the actively proliferating margin of the NVE and retinal ischemia below the NVE

A. Diabetic Retinopathy (continued)

Pars plana vitrectomy: Indications for vitrectomy:
- Tractional retinal detachment threatening the macula or showing progression
- Vitreous hemorrhage without resorption
- Recurrent vitreous hemorrhage
- Treatment-refractory neovascularization glaucoma
- Chronic macular edema without a positive effect after focal laser treatment

Prognosis. The following risk factors correlate positively with the start and progression of diabetic retinopathy.

Duration of the diabetes: The risks of development and progression of diabetic retinopathy increase with increasing duration of the diabetes. In type 1 diabetics, the incidence of diabetic retinopathy (NPDR and PDR) is 13%, with a disease duration of up to five years after diagnosis. The proportion of patients with diabetic retinopathy rises to 90% with a disease duration of 10–15 years. While the risk of PDR is 2% in type 2 diabetics with a disease duration of five years, this proportion increases to 25% with a diabetes duration of 25 years or more.

Blood sugar: Numerous studies have confirmed the negative effect of insufficiently controlled blood sugar on the progression of diabetic retinopathy. In type 1 diabetics without visible retinal changes, strict blood sugar control by means of insulin therapy diminishes the risk of developing retinopathy by up to 75% compared to conventionally treated patients. In 50% of treated type 1 diabetics with existing retinopathy, this therapy was able to prevent progression of the retinopathy compared to the control group. It should be borne in mind that strict control of the blood sugar in the first 6–12 months can lead to progression of existing retinopathy as a side-effect. In type 2 diabetics, the development and progression of diabetic retinopathy are reduced by strict blood sugar control compared to control patients (conservative treatment group). As a result, the need for laser therapy is markedly reduced.

Other risk factors: Arterial hypertension, hyperlipidemia, nephropathy.

Differential diagnosis.

Ocular ischemic syndrome: Can occur unilaterally. The retinal arteries are narrowed, and ischemic retinal hemorrhages are seen typically in the mid-periphery of the retina. Rubeosis iridis and anterior chamber inflammation are not rare as initial findings. Prolonged arm-retina filling time on fluorescence angiography. Carotid Doppler ultrasound is a crucial investigation.

Branch vein occlusion: Sectoral distribution of the hemorrhages and retinal thickening. A dilated retinal vein can be seen in the affected area of the retina.

Hypertensive retinopathy: Superficial and flame-shaped retinal hemorrhages, especially at the posterior pole. Depending on the severity of the hypertension, soft exudates and papilledema can be visible.

Radiation retinopathy: Ischemic retinal hemorrhages in the mid-periphery. The history of previous radiotherapy (usually for uveal melanoma) is crucial for the diagnosis.

Pregnancy and diabetic retinopathy. Pregnancy is regarded as a risk factor for the development or progression of diabetic retinopathy. If NPDR (mild to moderate) is present at the start of the pregnancy, ophthalmological review in each trimester is recommended. If progression or a severe form of NPDR/PDR is found, panretinal laser photocoagulation and monthly follow-up are recommended.

Cataract and diabetic retinopathy. Following cataract extraction, diabetic retinopathy can increase. Prior to cataract extraction, adequate treatment of the retinopathy according to the criteria given above should be provided.

A. Diabetic Retinopathy

Table 1 Ophthalmological examination in diabetic patients

Type of diabetic retinopathy	Follow-up interval
No diabetic retinopathy	12 months
Mild or moderate NPDR without macular edema	6 months
Mild or moderate NPDR with macular edema	3 months
Severe NPDR	3 months
PDR	1 – 3 months

NPDR = nonproliferative diabetic retinopathy;
PDR = proliferative diabetic retinopathy

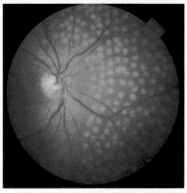

a Fresh exudates in the nasal half of the fundus with panretinal laser photocoagulation

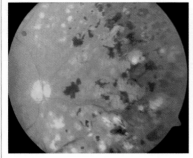

b Atrophic and partially pigmented laser spots following panretinal laser photocoagulation

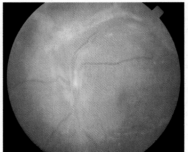

c PDR with marked traction at the posterior pole

Table 2 Laser photocoagulation of diabetic retinopathy

Stage of diabetic retinopathy	Technique	Laser spots
NPDR (severe)	Panretinal	2000 – 3000
PDR	Panretinal	2000 – 3000
CSME	Focal	Variable

NPDR = nonproliferative diabetic retinopathy;
PDR = proliferative diabetic retinopathy;
CSME = clinically significant macular edema

A. Fluorescence Angiography

In fluorescence angiography (FA) (**A**) a fluorescent dye is injected intravenously and its passage through the vessels in the optic fundus is recorded photographically. Upon irradiation of the dye in the vessels of the fundus with light of short wavelengths, light of longer wavelengths is emitted (fluorescence) . Using excitatory and blocking filters, which are incorporated in the radiation path of a fundus camera, the emitted light can be shown selectively and a fluorescence picture of the vascular structures of the optic fundus is produced.

The dyes used cannot pass through the walls of the retinal vessels (inner blood-retina barrier) or through the pigment epithelium (outer blood-retina barrier) when the fundus is normal, so leakage of dye is pathological. When interpreting the angiograms, a distinction has to be made between areas of increased fluorescence (hyperfluorescence) and those with diminished fluorescence (hypofluorescence). Hypofluorescence is caused by blockage (blood, pigment, etc.) or hypoperfusion, and hyperfluorescence by anomalous vessels, pigment epithelium atrophy (fenestration), or leakage.

Angiography with fluorescein (FA, Aa, b). FA is used particularly in macular diseases to demonstrate and classify choroidal neovascularization, and also to record perfusion disorders, the permeability of the retinal vessels and pigment epithelium, and pigment epithelium atrophy. Side-effects in the form of allergic reactions are rare. Angiography with indocyanine green (ICGA, Ac). In ICGA, the absorption and emission wavelengths are longer than in FA. In this infrared range, blockage of choroidal fluorescence by the pigment epithelium is slight. In addition, ICG binds more strongly to plasma proteins and thus leads to lower leakage activity than does fluorescein. This has advantages when imaging choroidal vessels and their pathologies, especially occult choroidal neovascularization, retinochoroidal anastomoses, and tumor vessels. Unlike fluorescein, ICG contains iodine.

B. Optical Coherence Tomography

Optical coherence tomography (OCT) (B) offers the possibility of noninvasive imaging of morphological structures in the fundus with high spatial resolution in the micrometer range. By means of reflection of coherent light, images of tissue structures are produced on the basis of their different light-scattering characteristics. The OCT picture of the healthy human retina shows two hyperreflective layers: the nerve fiber layer and, as the thickest band, the pigment epithelium-choriocapillary layer complex. OCT is used especially in the classification of macular holes, imaging of vitreoretinal tractions, pigment epithelium detachments, and macular edema, and to monitor treatment.

C. Multifocal Electroretinogram (MFERG)

The multifocal electroretinogram (MFERG) (**C**) allows objective measurement of the function of the photoreceptors and bipolar cells at the posterior pole and thus enables functional mapping of the macula. The diagnostic value of MFERG lies in early identification of Stargardt disease and toxic maculopathies. In addition, MFERG is an important supplement in the localization of unclear visual disorders.

D. Fundus-controlled Perimetry

Examinations of retinal function, with a simultaneous view of the fundus, are possible with a scanning laser ophthalmoscope (**D**). Kinetic perimetry and fixation can be measured along with automatic threshold perimetry. The direct correlation of morphology and function enables demonstration of small scotomas, which are particularly associated with macular diseases. Investigations of reading behavior with exact observation of fixation are also possible.

A. Fluorescence Angiography

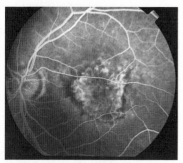

a Fluorescein angiogram: classical choroidal neovascularization; early phase

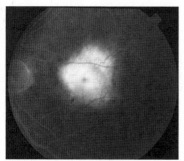

b Fluorescein angiogram: classical choroidal neovascularization; late phase

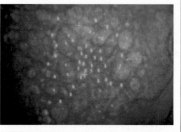

c Indocyanine green angiogram: choroidal neovascularization with feeder vessel from the choroidal vascular system

B. Optical Coherence Tomography

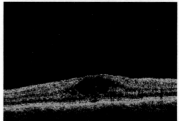

Cystoid macular edema

C. Multifocal Electroretinogram

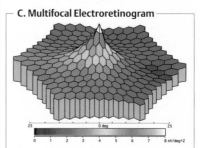

D. Fundus-controlled Perimetry

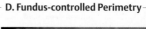

A. Age-related Changes

At a more advanced age, the macula shows a diminished oval light reflection and absent foveal reflection. The retinal pigment epithelium shows fine granulation, and a small number of small hard drusen can be observed, although these have no pathological significance (**Aa**, **b**).

B. Age-related Macular Degeneration (AMD)

Age-related macular degeneration (AMD) is now the most common cause of irreversible loss of central visual acuity and legal blindness in Western industrialized countries. Although there are usually no significant impairments of function in the early stage of AMD (**Ba**) when large drusen and pigment alterations are seen, a considerable loss of vision occurs in the late stages of the disease due to retinal pigment epithelium atrophy ("dry" AMD, **Bb**) or choroidal neovascularization ("wet" AMD, **Bc**).

Etiology/pathogenesis. A disorder in the metabolism of the retinal pigment epithelium leads to the formation of drusen (deposits between Bruch's membrane and the pigment epithelium). Ultimately, there is destruction of the retinal pigment epithelium, a chronic inflammatory process, and release of growth factors with the development of choroidal neovascularization (CNV). Apart from the confirmed age dependency, possible risk factors include female sex, nicotine abuse, intensive sun exposure, cardiovascular factors, and genetic components.

Epidemiology. The incidence of the late stages of AMD rises from 0.8 % in the 65- to 69-year-old age group to 6.8 % in the 80-years and older age group.

Clinical features. "Dry" AMD is characterized by increasing atrophy of the retinal pigment epithelium and the choriocapillary layer. Multiple small areas of atrophy develop: these are initially grouped around the fovea, and later extend into the fovea. The dry form usually develops slowly; as soon as the fovea is involved, there is a major reduction in vision. "Wet" AMD is characterized by the ingrowth of new choroidal vessels through Bruch's membrane into the subpigment epithelial and subretinal space. These vessels are fragile and are often associated with hemorrhages. Ultimately, CNV leads to extensive fibrous scarring of the macula (**Bd**). Metamorphopsia is the characteristic symptom. Clinically, CNV appears as a grayish subretinal lesion, surrounded by subretinal hemorrhages and edema.

Diagnosis. CNV can be imaged and classified by fluorescence angiography. Classical, occult, and mixed CNV pattern can be distinguished.

Differential diagnosis. Chronic recurrent central serous retinopathy, branch retinal vein occlusion of the macula, CNV in other diseases.

Treatment. The currently available therapeutic possibilities can usually only slow the progressive loss of function; there is so far no causal therapy. In "wet" AMD the treatment options depend on angiographic type of the CNV. Classical extrafoveal CNV can be treated by laser coagulation. When the CNV is subfoveal, photodynamic therapy is often used. Alternative treatment concepts include macula translocation, intravitreal injection of angiogenesis inhibitors, transpupillary thermotherapy, surgical excision of the CNV, and transplantation of pigment epithelium cells. Magnifying visual aids continue to be very important in both dry and wet AMD.

Prognosis. The spontaneous course of the various forms of AMD is very unfavorable. The ability to read is nearly always lost, but complete blindness is rare as the peripheral visual field is preserved. The five-year incidence of "wet" AMD in the second eye is 40 %.

A. Age-related Changes

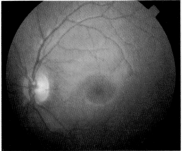

a Normal macular reflection

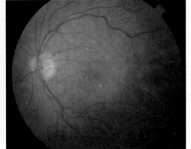

b Age-related changes of the macula: loss of the reflections, hard drusen

B. Age-related Macular Degeneration

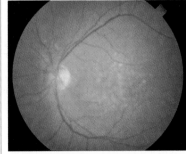

a Early stage of AMD with large confluent drusen

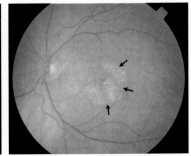

b Dry AMD with geographic atrophy

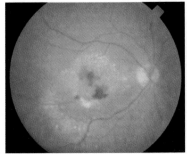

c Wet AMD with choroidal neovascularization

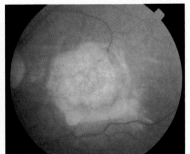

d Disciform scar

A. Central Serous Retinopathy (CSR)

Etiology/pathogenesis. A breakdown of the barrier in the region of the retinal pigment epithelium and the choriocapillary layer leads to a circumscribed serous retinal detachment.

Epidemiology. Mainly men in middle age; more rarely women.

Clinical features. The affected patients complain of a reduction in vision and metamorphopsia. The visual acuity can often be improved by providing glasses. If the vitreous is clear, a round to oval serous detachment of the retina can be seen in the fundus. Small detachments of the retinal pigment epithelium as well as atrophic changes can also be observed.

Diagnosis. The diagnosis is made by ophthalmoscopy, and can be confirmed by fluorescein angiography if necessary. Angiographically, one or more hot spots are seen, which appear like a smokestack initially and enlarge during the course of the fluorescein angiography, resulting in diffuse fluorescein leakage. Recurrent forms of the disease show multiple extensive areas of hyperfluorescence along with extensive atrophy of the retinal pigment epithelium.

Differential diagnosis. "Wet" AMD, optic disc pit.

Treatment. In most cases, spontaneous healing with resolution occurs within 2–6 months. If regression fails to occur or the condition is recurrent, focal laser coagulation can be considered.

Prognosis. The rate of recurrence is between 20% and 30%. When the condition is recurrent, extensive atrophy of the retinal pigment epithelium can occur with persistent visual impairment.

B. Epiretinal Gliosis (Macular Pucker)

Etiology/pathogenesis. Epiretinal membranes develop as a result of retinal vascular diseases or intraocular inflammation and following trauma and intraocular surgical procedures. The condition is usually idiopathic after vitreous hemorrhage.

Epidemiology. Common; correlation with age.

Clinical features. The clinical appearance is very variable, from an asymptomatic incidental finding to marked macular pucker with metamorphopsia and reduced vision. The macula initially shows glistening points, and later puckering with or without a visible membrane and distortion of the perimacular vessels (**Ba, b**).

Diagnosis. The diagnosis is essentially made on the basis of the funduscopy. Leakage from retinal vessels, possibly with the development of cystoid macular edema, can be observed on fluorescein angiography in the advanced stage.

Treatment. Pars plana vitrectomy with membrane peeling if the vision is reduced, or if the patient suffers from metamorphopsia.

C. Idiopathic Macular Hole

Etiology/pathogenesis. Tangential traction plays a central part in the development of a macular hole. If the vitreous is attached, detachment of the fovea occurs in stage I ("threatened" macular hole). Stage I can be reversed by vitreous detachment. In the course of the disease, there is usually an eccentrically located small tear of the retina (stage II). Ultimately, a fully formed macular hole develops (stage III) with or without an operculum . In stage IV, posterior vitreous detachment is also present (**Ca, b**).

Epidemiology. Women in the sixth to eighth decades of life are usually affected. Prevalence 0.05%. Bilateral in ca. 20%.

Clinical features. Besides the loss of vision, metamorphopsia and/or a central scotoma are reported. Stage I can be identified clinically by a yellow spot or yellow ring with attached vitreous limiting membrane. A complete retinal defect with yellow-white pigment deposits on the bottom of the hole and with elevation of the margins of the hole are characteristic in stage III.

Diagnosis. Optical coherence tomography (OCT) enables improved diagnosis of the early stages of the disease.

Differential diagnosis. Pseudoforamen in epiretinal gliosis, central serous retinopathy, cystoid macular edema.

Treatment. Pars plana vitrectomy with endotamponade for stages II–IV.

A. Central Serous Retinopathy

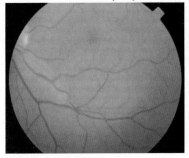

a Neurosensory edema

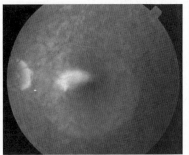

b Fluorescein angiogram with hot spot, smokestack phenomenon, and neurosensory edema

B. Epiretinal Gliosis (Macular Pucker)

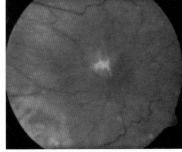

a Epiretinal gliosis (macular pucker) with distortion of the perimacular vessels

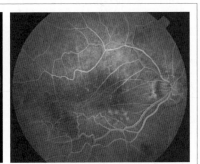

b Fluorescein angiography

C. Idiopathic Macular Hole

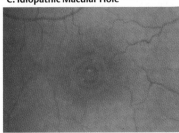

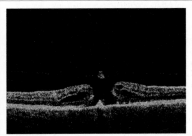

a and b Idiopathic macular hole (stage IV) with elevation of the hole margins and operculum on optical coherence tomography

A. Choroidal Folds

Etiology/pathogenesis. Choroidal folds arise when there is deformation of the globe wall due to a retrobulbar lesion or one within the globe wall, as well as in the case of hypotony.
Clinical features. The clinical and angiographic appearance is characterized by folds usually running horizontally (**A**).
Diagnosis. Choroidal folds are easily overlooked on ophthalmoscopy, but they are usually seen more clearly on fluorescein angiography.
Treatment. Treatment of the underlying disease.

B. Diseases with Choroidal Neovascularization (CNV)

Diseases that lead to inflammatory and degenerative changes in the macula or rupture of Bruch's membrane can cause a vasoproliferative process in which vessels from the choroid proliferate through Bruch's membrane under the retina. After an exudative phase with subretinal hemorrhages and neurosensory edema, this CNV undergoes a self-limiting scarring process (disciform scar) leading to metamorphopsia and considerable visual impairment (**B**).

C. Degenerative Myopia

Epidemiology. Higher incidence in women and in Asia.
Clinical features. The fundus usually appears quite pale with characteristic streaks at the posterior pole in which extended larger choroidal vessels are visible. Extensive chorioretinal atrophy (conus myopicus) is visible in the peripapillary region. Thinning of the sclera can lead to bulging of the ocular wall at the posterior pole (staphyloma), resulting in an increase in the myopia or in a circumscribed retinal detachment.
Ruptures in Bruch's membrane (lacquer cracks) are visible as yellowish atrophic streaks. These can lead to the development of CNV with severe visual loss. Finally, a pigmented scar remains, which is called Fuchs' spot (**B**).
Treatment. Photodynamic treatment of the CNV.

D. Angioid Streaks

Etiology/pathogenesis. A rupture develops in Bruch's membrane, which shows calcifying degeneration. Angioid streaks can occur in isolation or can be associated with a number of systemic diseases.
Clinical features. At the posterior pole, grayish to dark red "vessel-like" streaks, which run radially from the disk to the periphery, are seen (**D**). The retinal pigment epithelium over these tears is atrophic or demonstrates proliferation. Diffuse retinal pigment epitheliopathy with orange-colored granulation ("peau d'orange") at the posterior pole and peripapillary atrophy are also characteristic of this condition.
Diagnosis. Angioid streaks show hyperfluorescence on fluorescein angiography.
Differential diagnosis. Choroidal rupture.
Treatment. In the presence of CNV, treatment by laser coagulation or photodynamic therapy, depending on the location of the CNV.

E. Parafoveal Telangiectases

Etiology/pathogenesis. Not known.
Epidemiology. Rare, affects mainly patients in the fifth to sixth decades.
Clinical features. The ectatic capillaries are usually situated temporal to the fovea in a symmetric fashion. Should macular edema develop, metamorphopsia and a reduction in vision can occur.
Diagnosis. The telangiectases are demonstrated well by fluorescence angiography.
Differential diagnosis. Diabetic maculopathy.
Treatment. Because of the central position of the ectatic capillaries, laser coagulation is usually not possible; photodynamic therapy of the CNV.
Prognosis. Good prognosis for vision; the loss of vision occurs very slowly as long as no secondary CNV develops (**E**).

A. Choroidal Folds

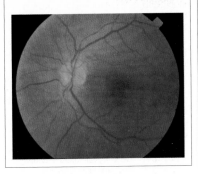

B. Diseases with Choroidal Neovascularization

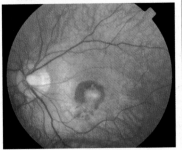

High myopia with choroidal neovascularization and subretinal hemorrhages (Fuchs spot)

Table 1 Diseases with choroidal neovascularization

- Age-related macular degeneration
- Myopia
- Angioid streaks
- Perifoveal telangiectases
- Traumatic choroidal rupture
- Hereditary drusen
- Vitelliform degeneration
- Disc drusen
- Multifocal choroiditis
- Presumed ocular histoplasmosis syndrome (POHS)
- Serpiginous choriopathy
- Birdshot chorioretinopathy
- Toxoplasmosis chorioretinopathy
- Choroidal coloboma
- Choroidal nevus
- Idiopathic

D. Angioid Streaks

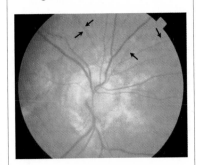

Table 2 Diseases with angioid streaks

- Pseudoxanthoma elasticum (Grönblad–Strandberg syndrome)
- Ehlers–Danlos syndrome
- Senile elastosis
- Paget disease
- Sickle cell anemia
- Thalassemia
- Acromegaly
- Idiopathic

E. Parafoveal Telangiectases

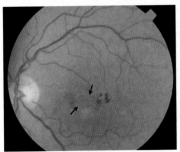

Perifoveal telangiectases with choroidal neovascularization (arrows)

A. White Dot Syndromes

Inflammatory diseases that preferentially affect the macula are collectively called "white dot" syndromes. They are characterized by multiple yellow-white spots at the posterior pole, and very often demonstrate the development of CNV as a secondary complication with an accompanying deterioration in vision.

B. Presumed Ocular Histoplasmosis Syndrome (OHS)

Etiology/pathogenesis. A disease in the USA which is ascribed in endemic regions to the fungus *Histoplasma capsulatum*; similar syndrome in Europe but without evidence of fungal infection.

Epidemiology. Healthy adults between the ages of 20 and 50 years.

Clinical features. Punched out, atrophic lesions ("histo" spots) in combination with peripapillary atrophy, peripheral pigmented striped lesions and noninflamed vitreous (**B**).

Prognosis. Tendency to recur; frequently CNV.

C. Multifocal Choroiditis

Epidemiology. Rare, usually young women.

Clinical features. At the posterior pole and in the mid-periphery of the retina, there are multiple whitish active spots and atrophic scars (**C**). Concomitant cellular vitreous infiltration distinguishes the condition from POHS.

Prognosis. Tendency to recur and to develop subretinal fibrosis; frequently CNV.

D. Punctate Internal Choriopathy (PIC)

Epidemiology. Rare, usually young women.

Clinical features. Usually bilateral disease with small indistinctly demarcated spots at the posterior pole, which develop simultaneously and heal with associated scarring (**D**).

Prognosis. Frequently CNV.

E. Multiple Evanescent White Dot Syndrome (MEWDS)

Epidemiology. Rare, usually young women.

Clinical features. There is usually unilateral loss of vision, which can be accompanied by enlargement of the blind spot. On funduscopy, the numerous very small white spots can be identified with difficulty in the outer retina (**E**). Orange granulation of the macular pigment is typical.

Diagnosis. Characteristic of this disease are its unilaterality and the fluorescence angiographic appearance with early hyperfluorescence of the spots, which are composed of numerous small hyperfluorescent dots.

Prognosis. Very good; the spots can resolve without scarring. Rarely CNV.

F. Acute Posterior Multifocal Placoid Pigment Epitheliopathy (APMPPE)

Epidemiology. Young adults, often following a viral infection.

Clinical features. The fundus appearance is characterized by bilateral, cream-colored lesions, which are usually larger than in the other "white dot" diseases (**F**). Concomitant mild vitritis is common. Systemic disease manifestations (erythema nodosum, cerebral vasculitis) are possible.

Diagnosis. The fluorescein angiographic appearance is indicative of the diagnosis. The acute lesions show early hypofluorescence and late hyperfluorescence.

Prognosis. Favorable spontaneous course with healing and mild scarring of the lesions. Rarely CNV.

G. Birdshot Chorioretinopathy

Epidemiology. Commences in middle age.

Clinical features. On funduscopy, medium-sized creamy-yellow choroidal infiltrates nasal to the optic disc and outside the vascular arcades with vitreous infiltration are seen. The characteristic depigmented scars develop in the subsequent course of the disease (**G**). Further deterioration of vision due to cystoid macular edema is possible.

Diagnosis. HLA-A29 association. Intraretinal leakage can be seen on fluorescence angiography.

Prognosis. Chronic recurrent course. Rarely CNV.

B. Presumed Ocular Histoplasmosis Syndrome (OHS)

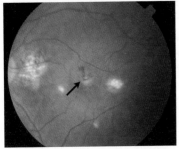

Presumed ocular histoplasmosis syndrome with choroidal neovascularization (arrow) and "histo" spots

C. Multifocal Choroiditis

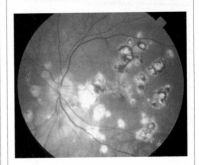

D. Punctate Inner Choroidopathy

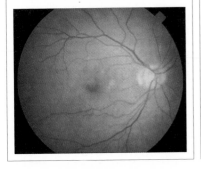

E. Multiple Evanescent White Dot Syndrome

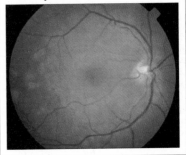

F. Acute Posterior Multifocal Placoid Pigment Epitheliopathy

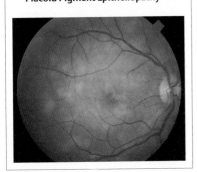

G. Birdshot Chorioretinopathy

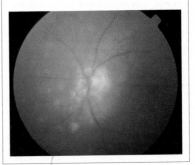

A. Stargardt Disease, Fundus Flavimaculatus

Etiology/pathogenesis. This is due to a mutation in the *ABCA4* gene. Inheritance is autosomal recessive.

Epidemiology. The most common macular dystrophy.

Clinical features. Typically Stargardt disease begins in the first to second decades of life with rapid deterioration of central vision, and the disease then progresses more slowly. In the fundus, a loss of the light reflection is found initially. An oval area of pigment epithelium atrophy develops, with an appearance that is reminiscent of hammered metal (**Aa**). Later in the course of the disease, this zone of atrophy can be surrounded by yellowish fishtail-shaped spots (fundus flavimaculatus), which can also occur in isolation.

Diagnosis. In the early stage of the disease, the multifocal electroretinogram (ERG) is indicative of the diagnosis (**Ab**). The electro-oculogram (EOG) is in the subnormal range. An extensive blockage of choroidal fluorescence is characteristic on fluorescence angiography.

Treatment. Optic rehabilitation.

Prognosis. Reduction in vision to 0.1 or worse.

B. Vitelliform Macular Dystrophy (Best Disease)

Etiology/pathogenesis. This is due to a mutation in the VMD2 gene. Inheritance is autosomal dominant.

Clinical features. Around the first to second decades of life, a characteristic prominent, yellow cystic lesion develops (vitelliform stage). Vision at this stage is usually not impaired. Later in the disease, the cyst content liquefies and sinks (pseudohypopyon, **Ba**), and the cyst ruptures (vitelliruptive stage, **Bb**). Finally, an atrophic macular scar develops, with increasing deterioration in vision.

Diagnosis. The EOG is diagnostic, demonstrating a reduced or abolished increase with increasing brightness, in the presence of a normal ERG.

Prognosis. Relatively good, many patients maintain reading vision in the better eye.

Treatment. Optic rehabilitation.

C. Cone Dystrophy

Etiology/pathogenesis. Cone dystrophy is the collective name for a heterogeneous group of diseases that are predominantly associated with abnormal function of the retinal cones. It often occurs sporadically or with autosomal dominant, autosomal recessive, and X-linked inheritance.

Clinical features. A slow reduction in vision with photophobia and a disorder of color vision manifests itself usually in the first two decades of life. Bull's eye maculopathy, in which a central island of intact pigment epithelium is surrounded by a ring-shaped zone of pigment epithelium atrophy, is a characteristic change on funduscopy (**C**). Commonly only a diffuse clumping of pigment in the region of the macula with temporal disk pallor is observed.

Diagnosis. An early disturbance in color vision is characteristic. The photopic ERG and the multifocal ERG are reduced; the EOG is unchanged.

Differential diagnosis. Rod-cone dystrophy, hereditary optic atrophy.

Treatment. Optic rehabilitation.

Prognosis. Reduction in vision to 0.1 or worse. D.

Pattern Dystrophy

Etiology/pathogenesis. Usually autosomal dominant inheritance.

Clinical features. Pattern dystrophies lead to only slight visual impairment in middle age.

Diagnosis. On fluorescence angiography, the typically butterfly-shaped, reticular, or granular "patterns" due to fenestration and blockade phenomena can be seen (**D**). The EOG can be subnormal, and the ERG is normal.

Prognosis. Good prognosis for vision; good vision is often preserved in one eye until an advanced age.

A. Stargardt Disease

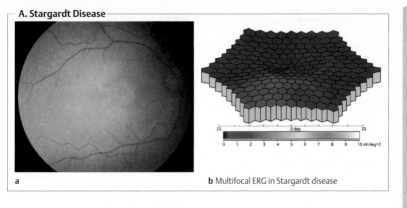

b Multifocal ERG in Stargardt disease

B. Best disease

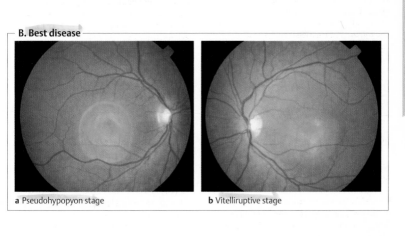

a Pseudohypopyon stage

b Vitelliruptive stage

C. Cone Dystrophy

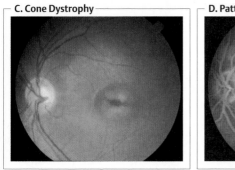

D. Pattern Dystrophy

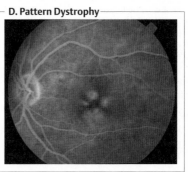

A. Berlin Edema, Commotio Retinae

Etiology/pathogenesis. After blunt injury to the globe, so-called Berlin edema can develop at the posterior pole indirectly as a result of a contre-coup effect. This is not retinal edema but more likely a fragmentation of the outer segments of the photoreceptors.

Clinical features. On funduscopy, a circumscribed region of gray-white discoloration of the retina can be observed (**Aa**). This can be accompanied by subretinal and intraretinal hemorrhages.

Treatment. Corticosteroids. Prognosis. Although there is a good tendency to regression, secondary changes such as gliosis, retinal pigment epithelium atrophy (**Ab**), or development of a macular hole can be induced. Relative and absolute scotomas can persist.

B. Choroidal rupture

Etiology/pathogenesis. After blunt injury to the globe, rupture of the choroid can develop indirectly as a result of a contre-coup mechanism.

Clinical features. After resorption of concomitant hemorrhages, the choroidal rupture is visible as a yellowish crescent-shaped line running concentrically around the disk (B).

Prognosis. During the further course of the condition, secondary changes such as epiretinal gliosis, retinal pigment epithelium atrophy, and choroidal neovascularization (CNV) can develop.

C. Purtscher Retinopathy

Etiology/pathogenesis. Purtscher retinopathy can lead to a disorder of the microcirculation as an indirect complication following abdominal or thoracic trauma. It has been suggested that the cause is a complex event consisting of traumatic vessel injury and formation of granulocyte aggregates.

Clinical features. The characteristic appearance is seen at the posterior pole with cotton-wool-like spots and intraretinal hemorrhages, grouped mainly around the disk.

Diagnosis. The capillary occlusions are visible on fluorescein angiography.

Differential diagnosis. Berlin edema, fat embolism from various causes.

Prognosis. Usually spontaneous recovery of vision.

D. Macular Hemorrhage, Valsalva Retinopathy

During a Valsalva maneuver, hemorrhages can occur beneath the internal limiting layer due to the increased venous pressure (**D**). Differential diagnosis. Hemorrhages due to coagulation disorders or hypoxia, hemorrhage from macroaneurysms.

Prognosis. Usually spontaneous resolution.

E. Solar Retinopathy

Etiology/pathogenesis. Light injury occurs due to phototoxic and thermal processes after looking directly at the sun or as a result of exposure to an operating microscope light.

Clinical features. The condition becomes apparent in the acute stage through an afterimage, blurred vision, and a central scotoma. On funduscopy, a small yellow-white foveal lesion can be observed, which regresses after a few weeks, leaving behind a small, reddish, sharply demarcated lamellar hole or pit (**E**).

Treatment. Corticosteroids.

F. Cystoid Macular Edema (CME, Irvine-Gass Syndrome)

Etiology/pathogenesis. Originally described following cataract extraction, CME can occur after any intraocular procedure. The prostaglandins released during intraoperative procedures are considered to be responsible for the development of edema.

Clinical features. Absent foveal reflection and cystoid breakup of the fovea with reduction in vision.

Diagnosis. Fluorescein angiography shows intraretinal leakage in the late phase from the parafoveal capillaries into the characteristic cysts (**F**). Optical coherence tomography (OCT).

Treatment. Corticosteroids; nonsteroidal anti-inflammatory drugs.

Prognosis. Although there is a good tendency to regression, a permanent loss of vision can occur.

A. Berlin Edema

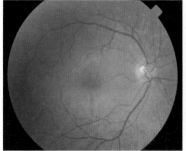

a Fresh Berlin edema

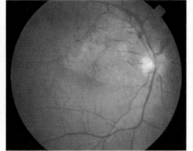

b Extended pigment epithelial atrophy following Berlin edema

B. Choroidal Rupture

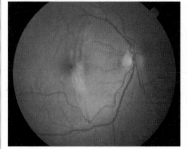

Fresh choroidal rupture

D. Macular Hemorrhage, Valsalva Retinopathy

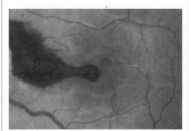

Macular hemorrhage following Valsalva maneuver

E. Solar Retinopathy

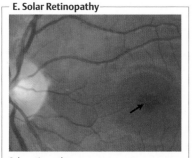

Solar retinopathy

F. Cystoid Macular Edema

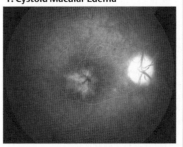

Fluorescein angiogram: cystoid macular edema

A. "Pseudopapilledema"

The most common congenital disk anomaly is an incidental finding of a prominent disk in **hyperopia** (**Ab**). It can be present unilaterally or bilaterally. There is no impairment of vision. In the fundus an often relatively small disk is found that is not cupped and that has an indistinct nasal or circular margin, however seldom more prominent than 3 diopters. The vessels are not concealed by edematous nerve tissue. The peripapillary zone is free from edema. Anomalous vessel origins from the arteries are often found with looping or trifurcations. If a spontaneous venous pulse can be observed, this argues against papilledema. No treatment is required. The prognosis is good, though there is an increased risk of anterior ischemic optic neuropathy (AION) (disk at risk). **Drusen** (**Ac**), which cause diagnostic difficulties particularly in children, are due to deposition of hyaline bodies, which become calcified during the course of life. The cause is a narrowing in the scleral canal, producing a disorder of axoplasmic flow. The condition is usually bilateral (66%). Since autosomal dominant inheritance is the rule, the parents should be examined if the diagnosis is unclear. There is no impairment of vision, but defects in the visual field corresponding to the course of nerve fibers can sometimes be seen. On ultrasound, calcified drusen are highly echoic with a subsequent acoustic shadow and can be seen even at low ultrasound power (**Ad**). Calcified drusen develop only by school age. Prominent disks are then seen, which are reminiscent of chronic papilledema but without edematous swelling of the peripapillary zone. With increasing age, the drusen come to the surface and are then visible as whitish shining bodies. Hemorrhages are possible in the superficial nerve fiber layer. During ophthalmoscopy, the light is shone beside the drusen, which makes them more clearly visible. The disk appears paler because of the drusen, which suggests atrophic papilledema or optic atrophy following anterior ischemic optic neuropathy. There is no treatment. The prognosis depends on the extent of the visual field defects, but these are usually not perceived subjectively. The risk of anterior ischemic optic neuropathy, like that of juxtapapillary retinal vein occlusion, is increased.

B. Disk Anomaly with Cupping

A **disk coloboma** (**Ba**) is an incomplete closure of the optic cup in the region of the optic nerve, usually inferonasally. The coloboma is unilateral or bilateral. It can continue into the retina and choroid and can also be observed in the anterior segments of the eye. Microphthalmos is possible. Spontaneous occurrence or autosomal dominant inheritance occur. Cranial midline defects of the face or skull such as hypertelorism, broad flat root of the nose, cleft lip, and basal encephalocele may be associated. Renal hypoplasia also occurs in combination with disk colobomas (papillorenal syndrome). The disk is enlarged and shows greater cupping below. Vision is affected to a varying degree. Serous macular detachment can occur as a rare complication. Because of the possible cerebral involvement, an MRI scan should be performed. There is no treatment except that of any amblyopia (e.g., due to anisometropia or squint) that is present.

Optic pits (**Bb**) consist of small, usually inferotemporal hollows in the disk, which correspond to hernias in the lamina cribrosa. They sometimes communicate with the subretinal space. They are unilateral, sporadic, and not associated with other systemic anomalies. Arched visual field defects are often seen depending on the location. Central visual acuity is normal unless serous macular detachment is present, which occurs in about half of cases in the course of life. The prognosis depends on the macular involvement.

A. "Pseudopapilledema"

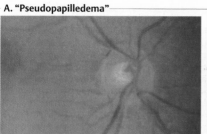

a Normal disk, right eye

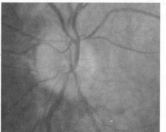

b Abnormal disk without cupping with indistinct margins in hyperopia, left eye

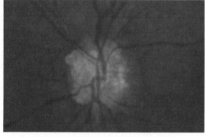

c Disk with drusen, left eye

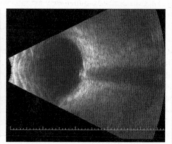

d Ultrasound with drusen

B. Disk Anomaly with Cupping

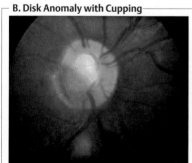

a Disk coloboma, left eye

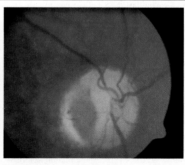

b Optic pit, temporoinferior, right eye

A. Disk Anomaly with Cupping (continued)

Tilted disk (**Aa**) is a congenital anomaly in which the optic nerve enters the globe obliquely. The disk appears oval and has a depression below and a relative elevation of the disk margin above. The vessels are often displaced nasally and scleroconus is visible below. The inferonasal fundus can be hypopigmented. If there is staphyloma in this region, the refraction differs from that of the macula. This leads to relative temporal scotomas in the visual field, which do not respect the midline. These scotomas disappear when refraction is corrected appropriately (usually myopic astigmatism). **Morning glory disk** (**Ab**) is a funnel-shaped cupped optic disc with a central depression and a circular change in the retinal pigment epithelium. It is usually unilateral. Vision is below 0.1 in 90 % of patients. The disk is well colored and enlarged. Centrally the disk is filled with glial tissue. The vessels divide too early. Serous retinal detachment can occur. Encephaloceles occur and must not be mistaken for tumors. Facial anomalies are possible. There is no therapeutic option. Deterioration in vision depends on the retinal involvement.

In **macrodisk** (**Ac**) the disk diameter is greater than normal. Major disk cupping is apparent, which according to the ISNT rule (inferior superior nasal temporal) has the thickest group of nerve fibers below and the thinnest one temporally, with no notching. Function is not impaired. Glaucoma must be considered in the differential diagnosis.

B. Disk Anomaly without Cupping

The more frequent **microdisk** is smaller than a normal disk with normal function and there is little or no cupping.

Optic nerve hypoplasia (**Ba**) is distinguished by the deficiency of nerve fibers, which leads to a varying degree of functional impairment. It can be unilateral or bilateral. The cause is unclear, but risk factors are young maternal age, anticonvulsant drugs, alcohol or hallucinogens in pregnancy, and maternal diabetes mellitus. Optic nerve hypoplasia due to diabetes is typically limited to the upper pole of the disk and is associated with corresponding inferior visual field defects. Vision and the visual fields are usually markedly impaired, but normal vision has also been described. When the hypoplasia is bilateral, nystagmus can be present depending on visual function, and a convergent squint is possible when it is unilateral. This can additionally lead to amblyopia, which is why occlusion therapy should be attempted in case of doubt. When the disk is clearly hypoplastic, an excessively small optic nerve is found in a normal scleral canal so that a pigmented double ring structure can be seen around the optic nerve. Disk photography is useful to compare the sizes of the two disks. Since optic nerve hypoplasia can be associated with cerebral malformations, such as de **Morsier syndrome**, which is characterized by absence of the septum pellucidum, chiasm hypoplasia, and endocrine abnormalities, or with **occipital porencephaly**, MRI and endocrine investigations should be performed in these children. There is no therapeutic option. Deterioration is not to be expected. The very rare, unilateral or bilateral **optic aplasia** can be regarded as an extreme variant. In this, nerve fibers are entirely absent, and the affected eyes are blind.

Medullary fibers (**Bb**) are myelin-containing fibers beside or on the disk and in the peripheral retina. This harmless condition is found in ca. 1 % of the population.

In **Bergmeister's disk** the hyaloid artery has not regressed fully. A remnant runs from the disk as a white strand toward the back of the lens, where a white Mittendorf spot may be seen.

Melanocytomas (**Bc**) of the disk are deep black, prominent abnormalities in the region of the disk and extending beyond it. This is a benign melanocytic tumor.

A. Disk Anomaly with Cupping

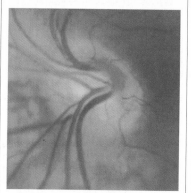

a Tilted disk, right eye

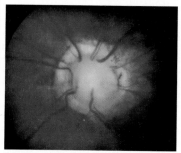

b Morning glory disk, right eye

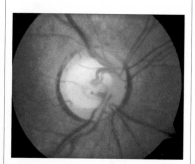

c Macrodisk, right eye

B. Disk Anomaly without Cupping

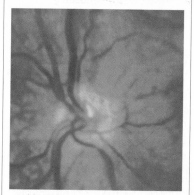

a Disk hypoplasia, left eye

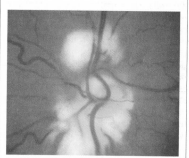

b Medullary fibers, left eye

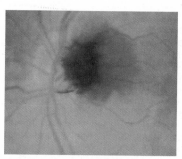

c Melanocytoma of the disk, left eye

A. Ischemic Optic Neuropathy

Nonarteritic anterior ischemic optic neuropathy (NAION, Aa is an infarction of the short ciliary arteries supplying the optic nerve. It is associated with sudden, painless loss of vision, which is usually noticed in the morning. It can worsen somewhat in the days following. Vision is between 1.0 and zero. In the visual field there are altitudinal nerve fiber defects, often in the lower half of the field. A relative pupillary afferent defect is always found. The disk margins are indistinct and prominent. There is diffuse or segmental disk swelling corresponding to the visual field defects (**Ab**). Hemorrhages at the disk margin and cottonwool spots occur. The patients are usually over 45 years old and often have cardiovascular or hemorheological risk factors. Small disks or disks with drusen have an increased risk of NAION. The other eye will be affected within 5 years in up to 20%. Within 6 to 12 weeks optic atrophy develops with segmental pallor of the disk in the affected area (**Ac**). There is no therapeutic option. Antiplatelet drugs are given prophylactically to protect the other eye. Investigation and treatment of risk factors is necessary.

An important differential diagnosis of NAION is arteritic AION. The cause of the optic nerve infarction is **Horton's giant cell arteritis**. The ophthalmological clinical findings and course do not differ from those of NAION but are usually more severe. Elderly patients are affected. The incidence among those over 70 year old is 27/100 000. In 10% of cases, temporary deteriorations in vision precede the event by 48 hours. Often, other symptoms can be elicited from the patients such as pain on mastication, headache, involuntary loss of appetite and general malaise. The pulseless temporal artery is thickened and nodular. The erythrocyte sedimentation rate (ESR) and C-reactive protein are usually markedly raised in these patients (**A, Table 1**). Since the risk for the other eye is very high, especially in the first 10 days after the initial event, high-dose steroid therapy must be instituted immediately, up to 1500 mg/day methylprednisolone i.v. for three to five days. This is followed by careful reduction (initially 1 mg/kg prednisolone) with ESR monitoring. A maintenance dose is given for approximately a year and, even after stopping the steroids, the ESR should be checked regularly as recurrences

are possible. An improvement in vision cannot be expected. Temporal artery biopsy is still possible a few days after the start of the steroid therapy. Only a minimal improvement in function can be expected in both forms of anterior ischemic optic neuropathy (AION).

Posterior ischemic optic neuropathy (PION) is a very rare variant of optic nerve infarction, in which painless loss of vision occurs without swelling of the disk becoming apparent. In this condition, also, there is always a relative pupillary afferent deficit and corresponding visual field defects. The disk becomes atrophic after 6–12 weeks. This form has been described with severe blood loss (when it is often bilateral) and in systemic diseases of the vascular system such as Wegener disease.

B. Radiation Optic Neuropathy

Radiation optic neuropathy can occur 6–9 months after irradiation of the paranasal sinuses, the nasopharynx, or the middle cranial fossa with a cumulative radiation dose usually above 6000 cGy and a daily fractionated dose above 180 cGy. The critical threshold can be lower if the nerves have been damaged previously, in elderly patients, or in those with diabetes mellitus or arteriosclerosis. Pathophysiologically, there is damage to the vascular endothelium with consequent ischemia of the nerve tissue. The patient notices a deterioration in vision while the fundus appears unremarkable. There is a relative pupillary afferent defect and nerve fiber bundle deficits are found in the visual field. On MRI, contrast enhancement is seen in the affected area. A therapeutic trial of steroids and full heparinization can be attempted, with subsequent changeover to coumarin derivatives with PTT and INR monitoring.

A. Anterior Ischemic Optic Neuropathy (AION)

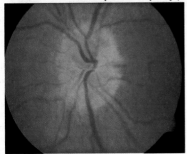

a NAION with obvious papilledema, left eye

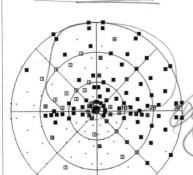

b Visual field in AION, left eye

Table 1 Symptoms of temporal arteritis
• Age over 70 years
• Pain on mastication
• Pain in the scalp region
• Pain in the shoulder girdle
• Loss of appetite and weight loss
• Fever
• Anemia
• Depression
• Marked loss of vision
• Can be bilateral
• Obvious disk pallor
• Tender, pulseless, nodular thickening of the temporal artery
• Raised erythrocyte sedimentation rate and C-reactive protein

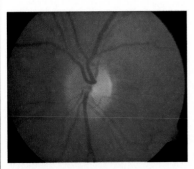

c Sectoral optic atrophy after NAION, left eye

Unilateral Optic Neuropathy

In patients with bilateral slow visual deterioration, abnormal color vision, and central or centrocecal scotomas, a hereditary, toxic, or malnutritional cause should be sought.

A. Hereditary Optic Neuropathy

The most common form of hereditary optic neuropathy is **autosomal dominant optic atrophy (ADOA)**. Mild symmetrical loss of vision occurs within the first decade of life. This is due to the destruction of retinal ganglion cells and their axons in the papillomacular bundle. The visual acuity is between 0.025 and 0.8. The ability to read is usually not lost. Temporal pallor is seen on funduscopy (**Aa**). Central or centrocecal scotomas are found in the visual fields (**Ab**). Deficits along the tritan axis in the panel D15 test are typical (**Ac**). Because both sides are affected equally, there is no relative pupillary afferent defect. Nystagmus can be present depending on the visual acuity and if the condition commences very early. As different degrees of severity within the family are possible, specific investigation of family members is necessary. The causative mutation is on chromosome 3 q. A molecular genetic test is available. There are no therapeutic possibilities. Over time, slight deterioration can occur but the ability to read is usually preserved.

Recessively inherited optic neuropathy occurs very rarely. The parents are usually consanguineous. Even at birth or in the first years of life, severe reduction in vision with pendular nystagmus and pale but otherwise normal disks and prominent retinal vessels are seen. However, electrophysiological investigations for the differential diagnosis of Leber congenital amaurosis are normal. Imaging of the chiasm region should always be performed to exclude compression in this area. Other systemic abnormalities are frequent. There is no therapeutic option.

Leber hereditary optic neuropathy (LHON, Ad) is a mitochondrial inherited optic neuropathy that is inherited from the mother. There are four known mitochondrial gene mutations: 11778 (50% of cases), 3460, 14484 and 14459. The mutated mitochondrial DNA cannot code the enzymes required for the respiratory chain and energy production is disturbed as a result. The retinal ganglion cells are affected selectively. The ratio of men to women is 8:1 with the 14484 mutation and 4:1 with the 11778 and 3460 mutations. The diagnosis is made biochemically from whole blood. However, the presence of a mutation does not signify clinical disease in the affected person (heteroplasmy). Before vision diminishes, telangiectases (**Ad**) at the disk can be observed in affected persons. Painless acute or subacute monocular deterioration in vision usually occurs between the 15th and 40th years of life. A relative pupillary afferent defect is seen. A central or centrocecal scotoma is seen in the visual field (**Ae**). The peripapillary telangiectases become more obvious, and the nerve fiber layer is thickened and slightly swollen. No leakage is seen on fluorescence angiography. Vision declines over days to weeks to 0.1 or worse. In the subsequent course the telangiectases disappear and the disk becomes diffusely pale (**Af**). Within weeks to months, the second eye follows. In 5% of the patients with the 11778 mutation, 22% with the 3460 mutation, and 37% with the 14484 mutation an improvement in vision can occur even years later. Systemic involvement with ataxia, peripheral neuropathy, or cardiac conduction disorders has been described. There is no therapeutic option. However, carriers should avoid tobacco and foodstuffs containing cyanide. Taking vitamins C and E, along with coenzyme Q, appears useful but there are no studies to confirm an effect.

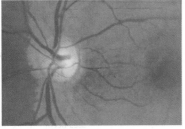

a Temporal pallor in autosomal dominant optic atrophy (ADOA), left eye

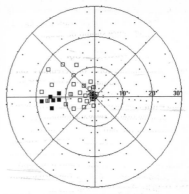

b Relative central scotoma in ADOA, left eye

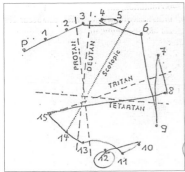

c Panel D15 color test (desaturated) in ADOA

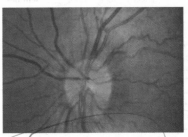

d Acute change in Leber hereditary optic neuropathy with vasodilatation and telangiectases, left eye

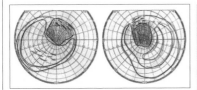

e Visual field with central scotoma in Leber hereditary optic atrophy

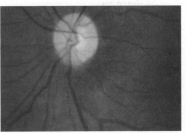

f Optic atrophy with long-standing Leber hereditary optic neuropathy, left eye

A. Toxic Optic Neuropathy

The toxic optic neuropathies (**A**, **Table 1**) affect the papillomacular bundle. They are associated with simultaneous binocular loss of vision and central or centrocecal scotomas (**Aa**). There is no relative pupillary afferent defect when both sides are affected equally. The deterioration in vision is often preceded by disturbances of color perception (**Ab**) and should be used for monitoring, particularly in the case of antituberculosis therapy. Examination should be performed prior to commencing treatment and repeated at regular intervals. If changes occur, the medication should be stopped. Avoidance of the causative toxin is the only possible treatment but is often not curative.

In **methanol optic neuropathy,** methanol is metabolized to formic acid, which leads to severe acidosis. Anoxia occurs in the area of the optic nerve, the basal ganglia, and parieto-occipital white matter. Vomiting, loss of consciousness, delirium, and parkinsonism occur in addition to the loss of vision. On ophthalmoscopy, the appearance is normal or there may be slight optic disc edema. After some time, the disk becomes pale. Therapeutically, the acidosis must be corrected first, but with severe intoxication the loss of vision, parkinsonism, and memory loss persist.

Ethambutol is used to treat tuberculosis. It leads to slowly progressive, bilateral optic neuropathy. Here, too, the fibers of the papillomacular bundle are preferred, so that a central scotoma and poor color vision occur. Chiasm involvement with bitemporal hemianopia is possible. At a dose of 15–25 mg/kg the incidence is below 3%. However, caution is needed in patients with renal insufficiency. After 2–8 months a disturbance of color vision and loss of vision occur. Because of the binocular involvement, there is no relative pupillary afferent defect. At the start there are no visible changes on ophthalmoscopy. Visual evoked potentials can be helpful. If the medication is not stopped, further loss of vision and optic atrophy occur. If optic atrophy is already advanced, no further improvement can be expected even if the medication is stopped.

Isoniazid leads to similar symptoms as ethambutol, but in this case optic disc edema can be seen.

Tobacco-alcohol optic neuropathy (**Ac**) is a binocular, slowly progressive optic neuropathy in patients who consume large quantities of tobacco and alcohol and have no other cause of disease of the optic nerve. Tobacco leads to an accumulation of cyanide compounds. A low cobalamin (vitamin B12) level, which often occurs in alcoholics, can further increase this. Alcohol leads to direct neurotoxicity. A genetic predisposition and vitamin deficiency, particularly of the B complex, appear to be needed for this neurotoxicity. The optic neuropathy can be improved with thiamin and cobalamin replacement. However, intramuscular injection of vitamin B12 in the form of hydroxycobalamin should be employed as cyano compounds can lead to impairment of the respiratory chain (see above).

B. Malnutritional Optic Neuropathy

Most nutritional deficiency states that include optic neuropathy involve the vitamin B complex. Thiamin (B1) is a coenzyme involved in energy production in the breakdown of glucose to acetylcoenzyme A. Folic acid and vitamin B12 detoxify cyanide and formic acid, which interfere with mitochondrial metabolism. Megaloblastic anemia indicates such a deficiency. When there is a deficiency of these vitamins, bilateral visual deterioration with central or centrocecal scotomas occurs. Optic atrophy develops in the subsequent course. In vitamin B12 deficiency, other neuropathies can occur as well as the bilateral optic neuropathy. Such a deficiency arises in pernicious anemia, after gastrointestinal surgery, or in fish tapeworm infestations. Replacement of the deficiency can lead to a certain improvement in the optic neuropathy. Use of hydroxycobalamin intramuscularly should be ensured in this case also.

A. Toxic Optic Neuropathy

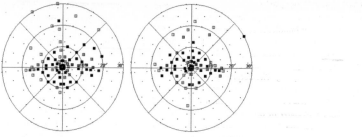

a Visual field in toxic optic neuropathy

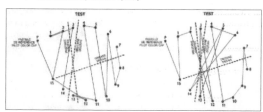

b Color vision in toxic optic neuropathy

Table 1 Most important causes of toxic optic neuropathy

- Ethambutol/myambutol
- Isoniazid
- Chloramphenicol
- Streptomycin
- Cytostatics
- Digitalis glycosides
- Penicillamine
- Tamoxifen
- Methanol
- Combination of tobacco and ethanol
- Lead

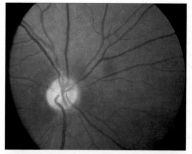

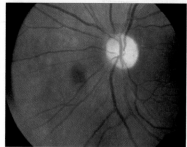

c Fundus appearance of tobacco–alcohol amblyopia

A. Typical Optic Neuritis

Optic neuritis is inflammation of the optic nerve from different causes. A rough classification into **typical** and **atypical** optic neuritis is made. Typical optic neuritis occurs idiopathically or in association with multiple sclerosis. In this case the myelin sheath is attacked. The picture of typical optic neuritis (**A**, **Table 1**) comprises unilateral deterioration of vision with pain on globe movement in patients between 15 and 45 years of age. Seventy percent of the patients are women. The vision fluctuates between normal and an absence of light perception. A relative pupillary afferent defect is always present unless the other eye has been previously damaged. Patients often report color desaturation. Nerve fiber bundle defects are found in the visual field. Temporary deterioration in vision in association with physical exertion (Uhthoff phenomenon) is also possible. Optic disc edema is found in only one-third of patients, which rarely is severe (papillitis). In most patients the disk is unremarkable (retrobulbar neuritis). Changes in the retina, choroid, or vitreous argue against typical optic neuritis. Deterioration in vision can still occur within the first week after the onset of the disease, and then slow improvement begins within another four weeks. Temporal optic nerve pallor rarely begins to develop after about five weeks. Delayed latency is found in the visual evoked potential (VEP) in optic neuritis. However, as this is also observed in other optic neuropathies, this is a very unreliable feature. When the clinical findings are clear, VEP is not needed to confirm the diagnosis. An MRI scan of the brain should be performed in all patients in order to estimate the risk of **multiple sclerosis (MS)**. Approximately 50% of patients with a first episode of optic neuritis show demyelination on MRI (**A**). If no foci of demyelination are found, the risk of developing MS within the next five years is 16% and is 22% at 10 years (**A**, **Table 2**). The risk at 10 years is 56% if there is one demyelination focus when the optic neuritis is diagnosed. If MS is suspected from the MRI scan, lumbar puncture can corroborate the diagnosis if increased immunoglobulins and oligoclonal bands are found. Typical optic neuritis is treated with an infusion of prednisolone 1000 mg/day for three days. In nearly all patients (80%) there is a marked improvement in vision within the first 30 days, but ultimate recovery can take up to six months. Ninety percent achieve a visual acuity above 0.8 within one year after the onset of the optic neuritis. The further prognosis depends on the frequency of the optic neuritis as this inflammation can recur, especially in MS.

B. Atypical Optic Neuritis

Atypical optic neuritis is much more commonly associated with other diseases than with MS. The symptoms do not correspond to those in **Table 1**. The patients are older or younger than in typical optic neuritis and there may be no pain on eye movement. On ophthalmoscopy, optic disc edema can often be found (papillitis). Investigations should then be performed with regard to **inflammatory** causes (**B**, **Table 3**). As there can be a specific cause, this investigation should also be done when there is a mixed picture of typical and atypical optic neuritis. The infectious causes include infectious meningitis/encephalitis, syphilis, toxoplasmosis, herpes simplex, herpes zoster, tuberculosis, borreliosis, bartonellosis, and bacterial or fungal sinusitis. Among the noninfectious causes, acute disseminated encephalomyelitis, Guillain-Barré syndrome, Crohn disease, ulcerative colitis, Reiter disease, Sjögren syndrome, Behçet disease, Wegener disease, lupus erythematosus, and sarcoidosis should be considered. As these are diseases that require treatment and the prognosis can often depend on early diagnosis and specific therapy, serological investigation is useful in atypical optic neuritis.

A. Typical Optic Neuritis

Table 1 Symptoms of typical optic neuritis

- Unilateral

- Pain on movement

- Color desaturation

- Afferent pupillary defect

- Age between 18 and 45 years

- Unremarkable or slightly edematous disk

- Begins within a week, then improves within four weeks

- No systemic disease apart from multiple sclerosis

Table 2 Risk of manifest multiple sclerosis (MS) according to MRI foci
(Optic Neuritis Study Group [multiple authors]. High- and low-risk profiles for the development of multiple sclerosis within 10 years after optic neuritis: experience of the optic neuritis treatment trial. Arch Ophthalmol. 2003) Jul;121(7): 944–9.

Number of demyelination foci on MRI	MS risk in the next 5 years	MS risk in the next 10 years
0	16%	22%
≥ 1		56%
≥ 3	51%	
Total	30%	38%

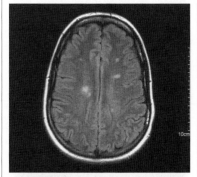

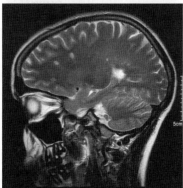

MRI scan in patient with typical MS foci of demyelination close to the medullary center of the cerebellum

B. Atypical Optic Neuritis

Table 3 Causes of atypical optic neuritis

Infectious	– Infectious meningitis/encephalitis – Syphilis – Toxoplasmosis – Herpes simplex, herpes zoster – Tuberculosis – Borreliosis – Bartonellosis – Bacterial sinusitis – Fungal sinusitis
Immuno-logical	– Postviral – Postvaccinal – Acute disseminated encephalomyelitis – Guillain–Barré syndrome – Posterior uveitis – Retinitis – Crohn disease – Ulcerative colitis – Sjögren syndrome – Behçet disease – Wegener disease – Lupus erythematosus – Infectious optic neuritis – Sarcoidosis

The optic nerve is involved in 0.5–5 % of closed head injuries. A distinction is made between precanalicular, canalicular, and intracranial optic nerve injuries (**Table 1**).

A. Precanalicular Injury

Because of its redundant course in the orbit, the intraorbital optic nerve is only rarely injured by trauma, as it is mobile to some extent. Nevertheless, injuries can occur especially due to direct injury (e. g., foreign body). In the worst case the nerve is avulsed from the globe, in which case the eye is blinded immediately. If bleeding does not prevent visualization, a gray hole is seen surrounded by a hematoma. There is no treatment. If the optic nerve is injured within one centimeter behind the globe, central retinal artery occlusion may also be seen. If the injury lies further posteriorly, no changes are seen in the fundus. Vision can deteriorate further after the injury due to compression as a result of a hematoma in the optic nerve sheath. Increased intraocular pressure and proptosis suggest compression by a hematoma outside the optic nerve sheath. If the intraocular pressure is over 40 mmHg, lateral canthotomy and cantholysis are indicated. When there is partial injury of the optic nerve, nerve fiber bundle defects are found in the visual field corresponding to the affected parts of the optic nerve. An afferent pupillary defect is present. After a few weeks, partial optic atrophy develops. There have been only isolated reports of optic nerve sheath fenestration for decompression of a hematoma located in the optic nerve sheath. There have also been only isolated reports of removal of foreign bodies compressing the optic nerve in the vicinity of its entry into the optic canal. Controlled studies are lacking.

B. Canalicular Injury

In closed head injuries, injuries of the optic nerve are usually canalicular. This type of injury is often found following blows to the head, even those not leading to loss of consciousness. A fracture of the sphenoid is found in only half of the cases; fractures of the optic canal are unusual and resulting injury of the optic nerve by bone fragments is rare. The pathomechanism is presumably ischemic damage after compression or shearing of the vessels supplying the optic nerve. Loss of vision occurs immediately and is only rarely progressive. Nerve fiber bundle defects are found in the visual field (**Ba**). The globe appears normal; only a relative pupillary afferent defect is found. After two to four weeks the optic atrophy (**Bb**) becomes visible. Treatment is controversial, and hitherto has usually consisted of high-dose steroids and/or decompression of the optic canal. However, up to 57 % of functional deficits improve spontaneously. High-dose steroid therapy is based on the results of therapy in spinal injuries. Surgical decompression of the optic canal can be performed transcranially or transethmoidally. The only prospective, nonrandomized study to compare the different treatment modalities in canalicular optic nerve injury-observation, high-dose therapy with 100–5400 mg/day methylprednisolone, and surgical decompression of the optic nerve canal-found no positive effect of steroid therapy or surgical therapy compared to observation alone. As a result, a recommendation on treatment cannot be given. Decompression of the optic nerve canal can be attempted if there is progressive deterioration in visual acuity.

C. Intracranial Injury

As a result of the sudden movement of the brain with severe blows to the head, axonal shearing of the intracranial part of the optic nerve can occur (similar to that which occurs with intracanalicular injury). Usually there is loss of consciousness. There is often a relative pupillary afferent defect with an unremarkable fundus. Optic atrophy develops after several weeks.

Table 1   Comparison of precanalicular, canalicular, and intracranial optic nerve injury

Site of injury	Mechanism	Treatment
Precanalicular	Direct effect	None; if necessary optic sheath fenestration, lateral canthotomy, cantholysis
Intracanalicular	Indirect damage due to acceleration movement	None; if necessary surgical decompression if progressive deterioration
Intracranial	Indirect damage due to acceleration movement	None

B. Canalicular Injury

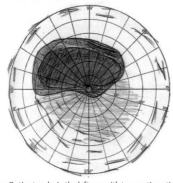

a Optic atrophy in the left eye with traumatic optic neuropathy

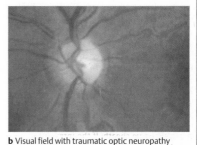

b Visual field with traumatic optic neuropathy

A. Compressive Optic Neuropathy

Up to 20% of brain tumors are situated in the region of the chiasm and so lead to alterations in the optic nerve. The prevalence of certain tumors changes with age. Pilocytic astrocytomas predominate in children. Gliomas indicate neurofibromatosis. Meningiomas occur more often in middle age. In old age, glioblastomas and metastases must be considered (**A**, **Table 1**). Since the only symptoms may be ophthalmological, the possibility of a brain tumor should always be considered. The visual acuity, relative pupillary afferent defect, visual field of both eyes, color desaturation, motility, and fundus appearance must be examined and the sides compared. If a tumor is suspected, imaging-MRI if possible-is urgently required.

Prechiasmatic tumor. When the optic nerve is damaged by compression, the presentation varies from patient to patient. The visual acuity and visual field can remain normal or be only slightly impaired for a long time with compression. A relative pupillary afferent defect is a very sensitive sign. If the tumor is in the orbit, exophthalmos, chemosis, motility, and sensation disorders and retinal folds are associated. When it is located in the apex of the orbit, chronic papilledema is possible (**Aa**). The disk can appear normal if the optic atrophy has not yet reached the disk; with slow growth, the disk can appear pale initially. Optociliary shunt vessels are possible (**Ab**). In the visual field, nerve fiber bundle defects can be anticipated. In the optic canal, the defects are nonspecific. The closer to the chiasm the tumor is located, the more the defect is oriented to the vertical midline. When there is a marked visual field defect of one eye and coinvolvement of the temporal visual field of the other eye (anterior junction lesion), a location close to the chiasm can be assumed. Slowly growing meningiomas can easily be mistaken for normal-pressure glaucoma. A tumor must be excluded with chronically progressive visual deterioration. These tumors may be difficult to diagnose, particularly with small meningiomas in the optic canal, and diagnosis is often possible only after repeating the MRI scan several times (**Ac**).

Chiasmatic tumor. Chiasmatic tumor presents with bilateral optic atrophy, which is often not symmetrical. Bitemporal defects are typical in hypophyseal adenomas but they do not have to be distributed equally (**Ad**, **e**).

Postchiasmatic tumors. Tumors in the optic tract are distinguished by homonymous, slightly symmetrical visual field defects with a relative afferent pupillary defect on the side of the temporal visual field defect, and asymmetric optic atrophy is common. The optic atrophy is in the form of horizontal bands on the side opposite to the lesion and is more marked temporally on the ipsilateral side. Neurological focal signs are possible.

Therapeutic possibilities. Therapy consists of irradiation or surgical removal of the tumors. A reduction in size can be achieved with bromocriptine only in the case of some hypophyseal adenomas. Close monitoring of these adenomas is required during pregnancy as they then have a tendency to growth. In the case of primarily inoperable tumors, radiation is given if possible. Gliomas in children are treated only if there is a tendency to growth. Radiation can be given over the age of 5 years. Halting of tumor growth is also attempted with chemotherapy. In all patients, regular visual field monitoring is indicated for prompt identification of recurrences.

B. Infiltrative Optic Neuropathy

Infiltration of the optic nerve occurs with carcinomas, lymphomas, leukemia, or intraorbital inflammation. The patients notice a deterioration in vision. The disk is normal or edematous. Imaging and possibly lumbar puncture may aid in diagnosis. Steroids are helpful therapeutically (1 mg/kg). With bacterial causes, antibiotic treatment is given initially. Optic neuritis must be considered in the differential diagnosis.

A. Compressive Optic Neuropathy

Table 1 Summary of tumors of the pregeniculate optic pathway

Arten
– Pilocytic astrocytoma (optic glioma)
– Schwannoma
– Cavernous hemangioma, meningioma
– Hypophyseal adenoma
– Craniopharyngioma
– Metastases (depending on primary tumor)

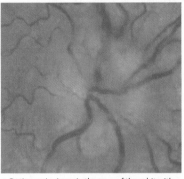

a Optic meningioma in the apex of the orbit with chronic optic disk edema, right eye

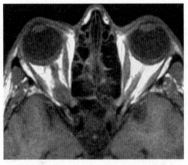

c MRI of an optic nerve sheath meningioma

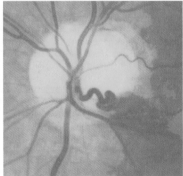

b Optic meningioma with disk pallor and dilated opticociliary shunt vessel, left eye

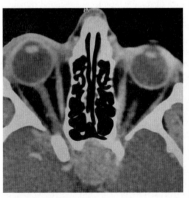

e CT of a hypophyseal adenoma

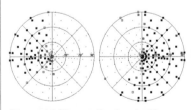

d Asymmetric bitemporal hemianopia with hypophyseal adenoma

A. Papilledema

When papilledema is bilateral in raised intracranial pressure, it is called **swollen (or choked) disks**. The axons are swollen. The raised intracranial pressure is transmitted along the optic sheath. In consequence, there is a disturbance of the axoplasmic flow at the lamina cribrosa. Swelling of the optic nerve and opacification of the retinal nerve fibers result. When the optic nerve is otherwise healthy, this phenomenon is **always** bilateral. When there is unilateral optic atrophy, the atrophic disk cannot swell and the papilledema is unilateral (Foster-Kennedy syndrome). Four stages are distinguished ophthalmologically: **early** papilledema is slightly hyperemic (**Aa**), the nerve fibers are only slightly opaque, the venous pulse is absent, and cupping can still be seen. With **fully developed** papilledema, hemorrhages and cottonwool spots are also found and the cupping has disappeared (**Ab**). The patient may notice transient blurring of vision. In chronic papilledema capillary ectasia is apparent, and the hemorrhages and exudates become fewer (**Ac**). Drusenlike bodies develop on the surface. Optociliary shunt vessels can develop. **Atrophic** papilledema is characterized by atrophy of the nerve fibers and corresponding visual field defects (**Ad**). Visual acuity is normal in acute papilledema and only alters late, except when macular edema with a star develops. In the visual field an enlarged blind spot is found (**Ae**). In the subsequent course, nerve fiber bundle defects are found initially nasally and inferiorly (**Af**).

Papilledema is a medical emergency. Imaging is indicated immediately, if possible MRI. If there is a space-occupying lesion, the further procedure is guided by the tumor entity. If a space-occupying lesion is not found and the ventricular system is not dilated, inflammatory and infiltrative causes must be excluded and the intracranial pressure measured by lumbar puncture. Changes in the cerebrospinal fluid are treated according to the cause. If the cerebrospinal fluid is normal and the intracranial pressure is raised, the cause is **pseudotumor cerebri (PTC)**. Apart from abducent nerve palsy, there may be no other neurological symptoms. In 25% of cases an empty sella is found on MRI. PTC is usually **idiopathic** (56–90%). Overweight women (8:1 compared to men) in the third decade of life are often affected. The incidence is 15/100 000. Idiopathic PTC is self-limiting but can recur. It is assumed that there is increased resistance of arachnoid cells to cerebrospinal fluid. The patients complain of headache, double vision, and blurring of vision. Visual field defects are found in 90% of patients. There is usually an enlarged blind spot, and concentric narrowing or nerve fiber bundle defects inferonasally. In addition to repeated lumbar punctures, treatment is with acetazolamide. Starting with 1 g/day, this can be increased up to 2 g/day and possibly more. Obese patients should lose weight. The surgical procedure depends on the symptoms; if the prescribed treatment is ineffective and the headaches persist, a ventriculoperitoneal shunt can be considered, and optic sheath fenestration with predominantly visual field defects. The prognosis is usually good. A persistent visual field defect after variable periods of time (weeks to years) is rare. Systemic hypertension, blurring of vision, multiple peripapillary hemorrhages, and advanced age are prognostically unfavorable with regard to the visual field.

Nonidiopathic PTC occurs with **sinus vein thrombosis**; use of exogenous substances such as tetracyclines, nalidixic acid, hypervitaminosis A, steroids, etc., or their withdrawal; and endocrinological disorders or systemic diseases such as lupus erythematosus, iron deficiency anemia, **systemic hypertension** with encephalopathy, uremia, or Lyme borreliosis. Nonidiopathic PTC must be treated according to the cause. Other causes of bilateral disk swelling are diabetes mellitus (incidental finding) and toxic or hereditary damage. However, in the latter, centrocecal scotomas are present.

A. Papilledema

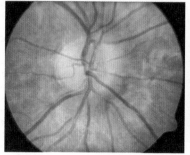

a Incipient papilledema, right eye

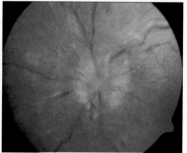

b Acute papilledema with hemorrhages and cotton wool spots, left eye

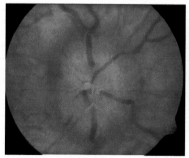

c Chronic papilledema, right eye

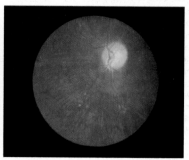

d Atrophic papilledema, left eye

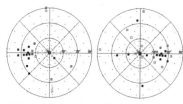

e Enlarged blind spot in papilledema

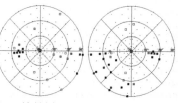

f Visual field defects inferonasally; pronounced and enlarged blind spot in papilledema

Papilledema

219

A. Optic Pathway

The optic pathway begins in the retina with the **photoreceptors** (ca. 125 million, first neurons). Still in the retina, the changeover to the second neurons, the **bipolar cells** (ca. 10 million) takes place. The impulse is then conducted through the **ganglion cells** (ca. 1.2 million) as far as the **lateral geniculate body** (LGB) (third neurons). In the LGB, changeover to the fourth neurons (ca. 5 million) takes place, which carry the impulse through the **optic radiation** to the **visual cortex**. Optic nerve. The axons of the ganglion cells run toward the disk in an arc in the temporal region of the retina, without crossing the horizontal raphe. Nasally they run straight toward the disk. After entering the disk, the peripheral nerve fibers remain on the outside of the optic nerve, while the fibers representing the central parts of the visual field run in the center of the optic nerve. If there is damage to the optic nerve during its orbital, intracanalicular, and intracranial course, unilateral nerve fiber bundle defects are found nasally in an arc (e. g., compressive) and temporally in a wedge shape (**A1**). A relative afferent pupillary defect (RAPD) is always seen on the affected side. After 6–12 weeks, optic atrophy is seen corresponding to the visual field defects. The second eye is not affected.

Anterior junction syndrome. Corresponding to the new order of the nerve fibers, visual field defects oriented to the vertical midline are demonstrated from damage to the prechiasmatic region. In the anterior junction syndrome there are marked defects in the visual field in one eye, while a deficit in the temporal half of the visual field of the other eye may be only suggested (**A2**). The cause lies in the fact that the nasal nerve fibers run in the same direction as the opposite optic nerve toward the opposite side before they reach the optic tract. Because of this asymmetry in the involvement of the eyes, RAPD can often be observed with lesions in this area.

Chiasm. Lesions in the chiasm are bilateral due to the crossing of the nasal nerve fibers to the opposite side, but are not symmetrical (**A3**). The RAPD is on the more severely affected side. Since it is limited on both sides by the carotids and cavernous sinus, by the hypophysis below, by the ethmoidal cells anteriorly, and by the floor of the third ventricle above, damage can

lead to blindness in both eyes due to the spatial narrowing and the high density of the visual information in this region. In general, patients with visual field defects that only suggest a vertical separation line should have immediate imaging.

Optic tract. Tract lesions are rare. They are characterized by homonymous visual field defects on the side opposite to the lesion, which are limited by a vertical midline. Postchiasmatically they are still asymmetrical because of the disorder of the nerve fibers. The more posterior the lesion in the optic pathway, the more symmetrical the homonymous defects become (**A4**). The RAPD can be on the side of the temporal defect. After weeks, asymmetrical optic atrophy is found bilaterally.

Lateral geniculate body (LGB). Wedge-shaped, homonymous visual field defects occur with lesions in the LGB. If the superior geniculate body is affected, the defect is directly above and below the horizontal midline (**A5**), while the two wedge-shaped defects are oriented to the upper and lower vertical midline with involvement of the inferior geniculate body (**A6**). Up to shortly after the LGB, an RAPD can be found on the side opposite the lesion.

Optic radiation. Following the LGB, the neurons fan out to the optic radiation. The inferior parts of the visual field are supplied by the superior parietal neurons (**A7**), the superior parts of the visual field by the inferior temporal neurons (**A8**). The far peripheral temporal crescent is represented anteriorly in Meyer's loop, which has no homonymous part in the opposite side (**A9** in 90° visual field). Lesions here are located in the temporal lobe at the anterior horn of the lateral ventricle. Visual cortex. The visual cortex is divided by the calcarine fissure into an upper and a lower part. The lower visual field is represented above and the upper visual field below the calcarine fissure. Half of the visual cortex represents the central 5° of the visual field (**A10**). The more peripheral parts of the visual field are represented more anteriorly (**A11**). The temporal crescent is represented furthest anteriorly.

A. Optic Pathway

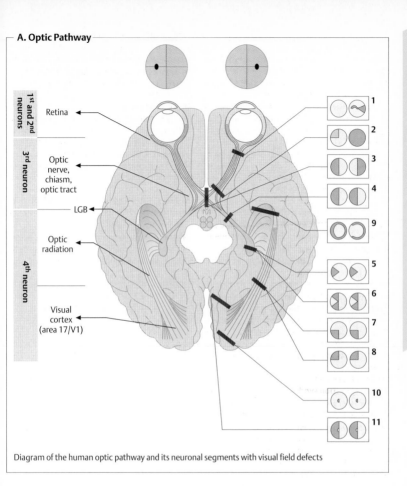

Diagram of the human optic pathway and its neuronal segments with visual field defects

A. Evidence of Causality

The medical literature constantly reports adverse ocular drug effects. It is certain that adverse drug effects on the eye are frequent even if a large number of them have not been adequately researched. Clear evidence of causality is lacking for many reported side-effects because they are very rare and thus only become apparent in isolated cases with long-term clinical use after a medication has been approved. However, knowledge of confirmed adverse side-effects of medications is undoubtedly one of the fundamental obligations of the clinical physician.

B. Changes in the Conjunctiva and Lids

The conjunctiva and lids can show numerous drug-induced changes:

- **Conjunctival hemorrhages,** e. g., due to anticoagulants, antiplatelet drugs, corticosteroids
- **Conjunctival hyperemia,** e. g., due to topically employed parasympatholytics (atropine), parasympathomimetics (pilocarpine), β-receptor blockers, prostaglandin analogues, cromoglycic acid
- **Toxic conjunctivitis,** e. g., due to topically and systemically employed antibiotics and eye drops containing preservatives
- **Conjunctivitis sicca,** e. g., systemically and topically employed (β-receptor blockers, eye drops containing preservatives (benzalkonium chloride)
- **Pseudomembranous conjunctivitis (Ba) in Stevens-Johnson syndrome/Lyell syndrome,** e. g., due to salicylates, antibiotics
- **Drug-induced ocular pemphigoid** (see below)
- **Pigmentation and deposits,** e. g., due to amiodarone, gentamicin, chloroquine, and derivatives
- **Necrosis of the conjunctiva,** e. g., due to anticoagulants
- **Allergic blepharoconjunctivitis (Bb),** produced by numerous topically and systemically administered drugs, particularly local mydriatics, miotics, and systemic antibiotics (especially sulfonamides)
- **Anesthesia of the conjunctiva,** due to topically employed (β-receptor blockers and nonsteroidal anti-inflammatory drugs
- **Lid edema, lid dermatitis,** e. g., due to gold preparations, synthetic retinoids
- **Photosensitivity reactions,** e. g., due to synthetic retinoids and nonsteroidal anti-inflammatory drugs
- **Depigmentation of the lids,** very rare, e. g., due to cytostatics (methotrexate)
- **Increased pigmentation of the lids,** e. g., due to topically employed prostaglandin derivatives in glaucoma therapy
- **Loss of lashes (madarosis),** e. g., due to cytostatics, amiodarone, chloroquine, and derivatives, acetazolamide, lithium, allopurinol, β-receptor blockers (topically)
- **Lash growth (Bc),** due to prostaglandin analogues in glaucoma therapy

C. Effects of Long-term Therapy with Antiglaucoma Drugs on the Conjunctiva and Lids

Topically employed antiglaucoma drugs lead to adverse effects particularly often because of their long-term use; these are caused not only by the drugs but often also by preservatives (usually benzalkonium chloride) (**C**, **Table 1**).

B. Changes in the Conjunctiva and Lids

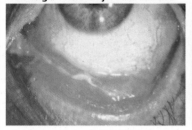

a Pseudomembranous conjunctivitis during gold therapy

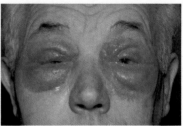

b Acute allergic blepharitis

C. Effects of Long-term Treatment with Antiglaucoma Drugs on the Conjunctiva and Lids

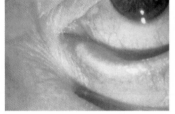

Occlusion of the inferior lacrimal punctum with use of miotics

c Lash growth with prostaglandin derivatives

Table 1

Beta-receptor blockers	Allergic blepharoconjunctivitis, conjunctival hyperemia*, corneo-conjunctival anesthesia*, loss of lashes (isolated cases), keratoconjunctivitis sicca*, contact lens intolerance, myasthenic syndrome (timolol), ocular pseudopemphigoid
Pilocarpine, carbachol	Allergic blepharoconjunctivitis, conjunctival hyperemia, ocular pseudopemphigoid, occlusion of tear ducts, superficial punctate keratitis, accommodation spasm*, narrowing of visual field, miosis*, transitory myopia*, vitreous hemorrhage, iris/ciliary body cysts, retinal detachment, pupillary block glaucoma, posterior synechiae
Prostaglandin analogues	Allergic blepharoconjunctivitis, conjunctival hyperemia*, lid margin pigmentation, lash growth and pigmentation*, iris pigmentation*
Carbonic anhydrase inhibitors	Allergic blepharoconjunctivitis, periorbital dermatitis, conjunctival hyperemia
Alpha-receptor agonists	Allergic blepharoconjunctivitis, periorbital dermatitis, conjunctival hyperemia, lid retraction (apraclonidine)

* = Common

A. Drug-induced Ocular Pemphigoid

Drug-induced ocular pemphigoid is rare and can be caused by topically or systemically administered drugs (**A**, **Table 1**). The pathogenesis is unclear. This may be an independent syndrome or a variant of classical ocular pemphigoid.

The symptoms include chronic conjunctival irritation and epiphora. The clinical picture in the **early stage** is characterized by chronic conjunctivitis and **shortening of the lower fornix**. In the late stage, the clinical picture corresponds to that of classical ocular pemphigoid (corneal pannus, development of symblephara, restricted motility). The diagnosis is based on the history, clinical picture, and immunohistological testing of a conjunctival biopsy. On immunohistochemistry, deposits of immunoglobulins (usually IgG) can characteristically be found on the basement membrane of the conjunctival epithelium but more seldom than in classical pemphigoid.

If drug-induced pemphigoid is suspected, the treatment consists primarily of stopping the suspected causative agents. This should be followed by close monitoring. If there is progression despite cessation of treatment, systemic immunosuppression is indicated as in classical pemphigoid (dapsone, mycophenolate mofetil). The prognosis is better than in classical ocular pemphigoid. The process often comes to a halt when the causative agents are discontinued.

B. Changes in the Cornea

Numerous medications can lead to degeneration and deposits in the cornea (**B**, **Table 2**). **Amiodarone** is the most common cause of cornea verticillata (whorl-shaped corneal degeneration, vortex keratopathy, **Ba**). At a dosage of 100–400 mg/day the first deposits are observed in the great majority of patients after only 1–4 months, and the full appearance is seen in practically all patients within 6–12 months. Symptoms (haloes) develop rarely. The clinical picture consists typically of bilateral, golden-brown, whorl-shaped lines of opacification within the corneal epithelium. Treatment is usually not required and the amiodarone does not have to be stopped because of vortex keratopathy. The corneal changes are completely reversible after the conclusion of therapy.

Cornea verticillata caused by **chloroquine** or **hydroxychloroquine** occurs in 30–75 % of those treated for several months. Initially, diffuse punctate deposits can often be seen, which subsequently change into the full picture of vortex keratopathy. Treatment of the corneal changes is not required. Vortex keratopathy during treatment with chloroquine or hydroxychloroquine without other ocular involvement is not a reason for ending the treatment. However, the dose should be reviewed as the keratopathy can also be a sign of overdosage. Examination and monitoring of retinal function are more critical as retinal involvement can lead to irreversible loss of vision.

Corneal changes such as superficial punctate keratitis, corneal erosion, and ulcer can be the direct or indirect consequence of medication use (**Bb**). Direct toxic corneal damage with topical use depends on the dose and toxicity of the substance, and, in the case of systemic administration, arises additionally from its secretion in tear fluid. Topical agents include neomycin, antiviral agents, benzalkonium chloride, corticosteroids, and the cytostatics 5-fluorouracil and mitomycin C, which are used topically in the course of glaucoma operations. The abuse of superficial anesthetics after corneal injury can lead to massive corneal damage. Production of lagophthalmos after periocular injection of botulinum toxin can induce exposure keratitis.

A. Drug-induced Ocular Pemphigoid

Table 1 Drugs producing pemphigoid

- With systemic use
  - ACE inhibitors: captopril, enalapril
  - Antibiotics: rifampicin, sulfonamides
  - Beta-receptor blockers: propranolol
  - Chemotherapeutic agent: sulfadiazine

- With topical use
  - Beta-receptor blockers: betaxolol, carteolol, levobunolol, metipranolol, pindolol, timolol
  - Preservatives: benzalkonium chloride
  - Miotics: carbachol, pilocarpine
  - Sympathomimetics: dipivefrine, epinephrine
  - Antiviral drugs: idoxuridine, trifluridine, vidarabine

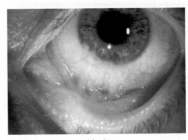

Fornix shortening/symblephara

B. Changes in the Cornea

Table 2 Drugs producing corneal degeneration and deposits

	Drug	Characteristics
Vortex keratopathy	Amiodarone	Common, reversible after cessation of treatment
	Atavaquone	Isolated case
	Chloroquine and derivatives	Common, reversible after cessation of treatment
	Indomethacin	Rare with long-term treatment, reversible
Pigmentation/deposits (without vortex keratopathy)	Amantadine	Rare, reversible after cessation of treatment
	Chlorpromazine	Common with long-term treatment, reversible after cessation of treatment
	Ciprofloxacin, norfloxacin (local)	Isolated reports during treatment of keratitis, reversible
	Gold	Common with long-term treatment and total dose > 1 g, reversible after stopping
	Isotretinoin	Incidence not known, reversible
Bandlike degeneration	Prednisolone phosphate eye drops	Isolated cases with preexisting corneal surface defects
	Vitamin D	Signs of vitamin D intoxication

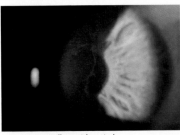

a Cornea verticillata with amiodarone

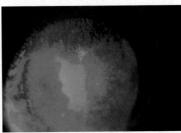

b Corneal erosion with 5-fluorouracil

A. Corticosteroid-induced Ocular Hypertension/Steroid Glaucoma

Steroid glaucoma is a secondary open-angle glaucoma.

Etiology/pathogenesis. The rise in the intraocular pressure is due to an increase in trabecular outflow resistance as a result of biochemical and morphological changes in the trabecular meshwork cells. These can include changes in cell morphology (cytoskeleton, cell nucleus size), in cell function (phagocytosis, cell migration, cell proliferation), and in the composition of the extracellular matrix. However, the precise pathogenesis is still unclear.

Epidemiology. Approximately 5% of the healthy general population show a marked rise in intraocular pressure within 4–6 weeks of local corticosteroid administration (so-called high responders; **A**, **Table 1**). In addition to individual sensitivity, the likelihood of a rise in intraocular pressure is influenced by additional risk factors (**A**, **Table 2**) and by the duration, route of administration, dosage, and potency of the corticosteroid.

Clinical features. An increase in pressure occurs at the earliest 1–2 weeks after the start of the corticosteroid therapy, up to months to years later with continued therapy. In early childhood, a clinical picture similar to that of congenital/juvenile glaucoma can develop (see Chapter 12). In late childhood and adulthood, the clinical picture is then similar to that of primary chronic open-angle glaucoma, i.e., usually an asymptomatic insidious start with a noninflamed eye, increased intraocular pressure, and possibly disk and visual field changes (**A**). **Diagnosis.** The diagnosis is made from a careful history of previous or current use of corticosteroids along with the usual investigations in glaucoma (see Chapter 12). Other visible corticosteroid-induced changes (e.g., secondary cataract) can support the diagnosis.

Treatment. Treatment consists mainly of stopping the corticosteroid therapy if at all possible. Otherwise it is similar to that of primary chronic open-angle glaucoma.

Prognosis. Prognosis is good because normalization of the intraocular pressure usually occurs within a few weeks after stopping the corticosteroid therapy. In many patients, therefore, steroids cause transient ocular hypertension without lasting optic nerve damage. If it does occur, glaucomatous optic neuropathy is irreversible.

B. Other Forms of Drug-induced Increase in the Intraocular Pressure

Mydriatics/cycloplegics rarely cause acute angle-closure glaucoma. This occurs in eyes with preexisting narrow anterior chamber angles. The risk of a rise in pressure is much higher when glaucoma has already been diagnosed: >30% of patients with primary chronic open-angle glaucoma show a rise in the intraocular pressure of >5 mmHg with use of mydriatics.

Many **psychotropic medications** can also cause acute angle-closure glaucoma because of their simultaneous anticholinergic effect. This is a very rare side-effect. A range of different drugs (especially **sulfonamides** and derivatives) can in very rare cases cause an acute rise in intraocular pressure through anterior displacement of the iris-lens diaphragm (angle-closure glaucoma without pupillary block) because of ciliary body edema. Secondary glaucoma as a result of an intraocular hemorrhage during treatment with **coumarin derivatives** is an extremely serious side-effect (**Ba**, **b**). Patients with exudative age-related macular degeneration are particularly predisposed. The condition is very difficult to control therapeutically and leads to loss of the eye or to blindness in >50% of cases.

Paradoxical rises in pressure can occur as a result of topical administration of **antiglaucoma agents**. These include an increase in pupillary block due to pilocarpine or a rise in pressure during combined therapy with prostaglandin derivatives.

A. Corticosteroid-induced Ocular Hypertension/Steroid Glaucoma

Table 1 Steroid responders in the healthy general population with local treatment with potent corticosteroids after Armaly (1965) and Becker (1965)

Eye drops	Low responders (%)	Intermediate responders (%)	High responders (%)
Dexamethasone 0,1 % (4 weeks)[1]	66 IOD ↑ < 6 mmHg	29 IOD ↑ = 6 – 15 mmHg	5 IOD ↑ > 15 mmHg
Betamethason (6 weeks)[2]	58 IOD < 20 mmHg	36 IOD = 20 – 31 mmHg	6 IOD > 31 mmHg

IOD = intraocular pressure, IOD ↑ = increase of IOP

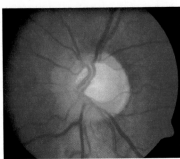

Glaucomatous disk cupping

Table 2 Predisposing ocular and general diseases that increase the risk of corticosteroid-induced rise in intraocular pressure

- Primary chronic open-angle glaucoma
- First-degree relatives of patients with primary chronic open-angle glaucoma
- Angle recession glaucoma (traumatic glaucoma)
- High myopia
- Diabetes mellitus
- Connective-tissue diseases (especially rheumatoid arthritis)
- Cushing syndrome

B. Other Forms of Drug-induced Increase in the Intraocular Pressure

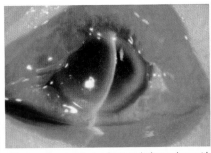

a Massive subconjunctival and intraocular hemorrhage with anticoagulants

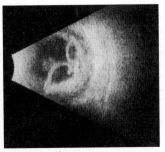

b Massive subretinal hemorrhage and exudative detachment during anticoagulant treatment

A. Drug-induced Cataract

The number of medications known to produce cataract in clinical use is limited (**A**, **Table 1**). Undoubtedly, **glucocorticosteroid-induced cataract (Aa)** is by far the most common drug-induced lens opacity overall and is also the most common ocular complication of such therapy. The precise pathogenesis is not known. The lens opacity can be produced by any form of steroid therapy (oral, topical, inhalation). With oral administration of 10 mg prednisolone equivalent daily for more than a year there is a relatively high risk of cataract development, but there is no safe threshold dose for avoiding it. Children's lenses are more sensitive in principle than those of adults but are believed to have a limited capacity for regression of the opacities. Clinically there is typically a posterior capsule opacity of variable severity, which can cause marked glare sensitivity and myopia to develop along with the deterioration in vision. In advanced cases there is complete opacification of the full thickness of the lens, which then does not differ morphologically from a senile cataract. Cataract extraction can be performed without an increased risk of intraoperative and postoperative complications.

B. Changes in the Sclera

Drug side-effects in the sclera are very rare (bradytrophic metabolism). Episcleritis and scleritis have been described in conjunction with bisphosphonate use (palmidronic acid) and after topical use of mitomycin C; scleral atrophy with mitomycin C and corticosteroids; orange discoloration of the sclera with systemic administration of rifabutin; and scleral calcification with vitamin D overdose.

C. Changes in the Lacrimal Apparatus

The keratoconjunctivitis sicca that can be produced by numerous topically or systemically administered medications is due in many cases to **hyposecretion of the lacrimal gland**, which can be attributed, for example, to an anticholinergic component of the effect (psychotropic drugs) or to direct alterations in the tissues of the lacrimal gland (lipofuscin deposition due to amiodarone). **Stenosis of the lacrimal ducts** can develop with systemic administration of quinacrine or 5-fluorouracil and with prolonged local therapy with antiglaucoma agents (parasympathomimetics, epinephrine) and antiviral drugs.

D. Changes in the Orbit and Ocular Muscles

Among the most important orbital changes during medication use are the rare spontaneous **hemorrhages**, which can be produced as a result of intravenous thrombolytic therapy with streptokinase, urokinase, and tissue plasminogen activator (TPA) and by various heparins. A possible cause of heparin-induced bleeding is IgG antibody-mediated thrombocytopenia, which should therefore always be excluded in every case.

A range of medications can lead to exophthalmos by affecting **thyroid metabolism** (antithyroid drugs, vitamin A, lithium). Oral long-term therapy with corticosteroids can lead to reversible exophthalmos by increasing the intraorbital fat tissue.

Numerous medications can lead in various ways to an impairment of the **ocular muscles**; these include ocular muscle palsies (e. g., botulinum toxin in essential blepharospasm), triggering of a myasthenic syndrome or deterioration of myasthenia (e. g., numerous antibiotics), total external ophthalmoplegia (e. g., amitriptyline), internuclear ophthalmoplegia (e. g., cimetidine), nystagmus (e. g., aminoglycosides, antiepileptic drugs), and oculogyric crisis (e. g., antidepressants).

A. Drug-induced Cataract

Table 1 Drugs confirmed to induce cataract in clinical use

Drug	Type of lens opacity	Dose-dependency, course
Amiodarone	Anterior, subcapsular, white-yellow opacities	Dose-dependent, in 50–60 % of patients on long-term treatment, not visually significant, cessation of treatment not necessary
Busulfan	Posterior subcapsular opacity, polychromatic reflexes	Dose-dependent in 10–30 % of patients
Chlorpromazine (**Ab**)	Yellow-brown central subcapsular deposits with isolated peripheral extensions	Only with long-term treatment for several years (cumulative dose > 500 g), in 40% at a dose of 300 mg/day for more than 3 years, not visually significant, cessation of treatment not necessary
Glucocorticosteroids	Unilateral or bilateral, posterior subcapsular opacity	Slowly progressive, no definite dose dependency
Gold salts	Chrysiasis lentis: fine granular yellowish deposits in the central anterior capsule and in the suture system of the lens	With long-term treatment and a cumulative dose > 2.5 g in over 50% of patients, no deterioration in vision, discontinuation of treatment not required
Methoxsalen/PUVA therapy	Anterior, subcapsular opacity	Lens opacities avoidable by wearing UV protective glasses on the day of irradiation

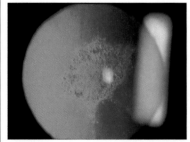

a Steroid cataract

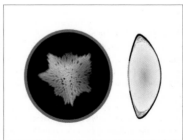

b Chlorpromazine-induced lens opacity

A. Changes in the Retina

The adrenergic drugs epinephrine and its pro-drug dipivefrine, which are rarely used today as **antiglaucoma agents**, are contraindicated in aphakic patients because they cause macular edema. There is no confirmed connection between the prostaglandin analogues also used topically in glaucoma therapy and the production of macular edema. However, close monitoring is recommended in aphakic/pseudophakic patients. The miotics pilocarpine and carbachol can very rarely cause rhegmatogenous retinal detachment, especially when there is preexisting retinal pathology. In patients with risk factors for retinal detachment, miotics should therefore be used cautiously.

Long-term use of **chloroquine** and **hydroxychloroquine** in the treatment of collagenoses and rheumatic diseases can lead to irreversible retinal damage. This side-effect is rare with average dosage (chloroquine 250 mg/day or less than 3.5–4.0 mg/kg/day; hydroxychloroquine 400 mg/day or less than 6.0–6.5 mg/kg/day) but is more commonly due to chloroquine. In the early stage, fine pigment changes of the macula are found, which are not yet associated with changes in visual acuity or the visual fields. In the late stage, marked pigment changes occur in the macular region (bull's eye maculopathy) with a reduction in visual acuity and visual field defects. The condition is not reversible even after stopping the treatment and can deteriorate further. Treatment consists of stopping the medication in consultation with the treating internist. In principle, patients on this treatment should be screened (vision, color vision, macular appearance) with a baseline examination and review every six months. The antiestrogen **tamoxifen**, which is used in the treatment of breast cancer, can (in up to 6 %) lead to yellow-white, partially reflective, intraretinal deposits with a preference for the macula, which can be associated with macular edema (**Aa**). A corresponding reduction in visual acuity can occur. In consultation with the treating oncologist, a reduction in dose or cessation of therapy should be encouraged.

Macular changes are known to occur with a range of other medications such as quinine, hydrochlorothiazide, indomethacin, or mitomycin C (hypotony maculopathy after glaucoma surgery). Patients with wet age-related macular degeneration in particular have a high risk of developing massive intraocular hemorrhage on anticoagulant therapy. Such an increased risk has not been confirmed for antiplatelet drugs.

The use of **interferon-alfa**, especially to treat chronic hepatitis B and C, can be associated with the development of retinal vascular changes (cottonwool spots, punctate hemorrhages, central retinal vein, branch retinal vein, and branch retinal artery occlusions) (**Ab**). The incidence and pathogenesis are unclear.

The **phenothiazines** thioridazine and fluphenazine can cause changes in the retinal pigment epithelium, which lead to a reduction in visual acuity and disorders of color perception and dark adaptation. Usually symptoms regress completely after conclusion of treatment. Six-month screening during treatment is recommended. The antiepileptic drug **vigabatrin**, used in severe forms of childhood epilepsy, frequently causes irreversible, concentric visual field defects (**Ac**). Ocular side-effects must be weighed against the benefit of treatment.

B. Changes in the Uveal Tract

A range of medications are suspected to be causes of **uveitis**. These include the topically used antiglaucoma agents metipranolol (β-receptor blocker), prostaglandin analogues, and (in glaucoma surgery) the cytostatics mitomycin C and 5-fluorouracil. The medications used systemically include bisphosphonates, quinine, rifabutin, sulfonamides, and vaccines. For the majority of the listed drugs, there is no confirmed association between administration of the medication and uveitis.

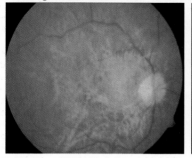

a Tamoxifen-induced retinopathy

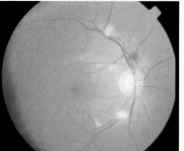

b α-Interferon-induced retinopathy

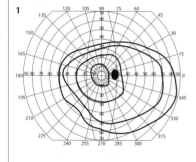

1

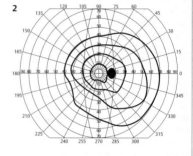

2

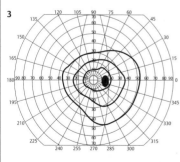

3

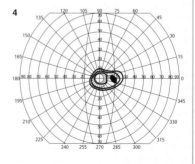

4

c Stage-dependent vigabatrin-induced visual field restriction (1, normal; 2, slight restriction; 3, moderate restriction; 4, severe restriction)

A. Changes in the Optic Nerve and Optic Pathway

The following drug-induced changes can be distinguished:

• Anterior ischemic optic neuropathy
• Optic neuritis-like neuropathy
• Papilledema/optic atrophy

Anterior ischemic optic neuropathy (AION) can rarely be caused by amiodarone, ergotamine, interferon alpha, and oral contraceptives. The extent of the reduction in vision is variable and, as in other forms of AION, it is usually irreversible. If **amiodarone-induced** AION occurs, cessation of treatment must be considered in order to avoid manifestation in the other eye. However, this depends on the often-vital indication for amiodarone therapy and must therefore be evaluated in each individual case. AION with the use of modern contraceptives can be classified as very rare.

Optic neuritis-like neuropathy is a drug-induced toxic neuropathy that resembles optic neuritis clinically and is associated with recovery of visual acuity if the causative medication is discontinued early. Besides numerous other medications, the tuberculostatic drug **ethambutol** should be mentioned in particular, which can cause an axial (reduction in vision, central scotoma, decreased green vision sensitivity) or paraxial optic neuropathy (peripheral or paracentral visual field defects, normal visual acuity, normal color vision) only days to a few weeks after the start of treatment (**Aa** and **b**). An examination of vision, the visual fields, and color vision should be performed within the first two weeks after the start of treatment and then continued at intervals of six weeks. If ocular changes are discovered early, there is a good prospect of a gradual regression of the changes after stopping the ethambutol treatment. If the treatment is continued, severe, irreversible damage to vision as a result of optic atrophy can be expected. Isoniazid, which is usually used in combination with ethambutol, also has a neurotoxic effect, but this appears to be much less than that of ethambutol.

Optic atrophy and optic neuritis-like neuropathy and also cortical blindness and homonymous hemianopia have also been described in conjunction with intra-arterial or intrathecal injection of cytostatics such as methotrexate, cisplatin, or carmustine. Cortical blindness and hemianopia have also been observed in isolated cases with the use of vinca alkaloids, interleukin 2, interferon alpha, tacrolimus, and cyclosporin A. The cause of the cortical blindness with cyclosporin A and tacrolimus is neurotoxically induced posterior leukoencephalopathy.

B. Changes in Pupillary Function, Refraction, and Accommodation

Undesirable pupil dilatation after systemic administration of medication is very rare and is due mainly to abuse (amphetamines) or overdosage (barbiturates, carbamazepine, phenothiazines, tricyclic antidepressants, chloroquine, quinine, clonidine). The parasympatholytics used topically for the purpose of mydriasis (atropine, tropicamide) additionally cause paralysis of accommodation that varies in duration. Pupil constriction is a side-effect observed in all glaucoma patients after the use of the direct parasympathomimetics pilocarpine and carbachol. This can cause additional visual field restriction. As well as the miosis, transitory myopia is the most common side-effect produced by **miotics** (duration of 2–3 hours with a single use). The cause is ciliary body spasm. Other medications (sulfonamides, carbonic anhydrase inhibitors) can rarely cause transitory myopia as a result of ciliary body edema (**B**). The side-effect is completely reversible within a few days after stopping the medication.

A. Changes in the Optic Nerve and Optic Pathway

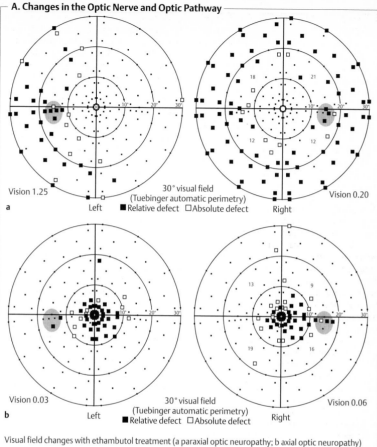

Vision 1.25

30° visual field
(Tuebinger automatic perimetry)

Left

Vision 0.20

Right

a ■ Relative defect □ Absolute defect

Vision 0.03

30° visual field
(Tuebinger automatic perimetry)

Left

Vision 0.06

Right

b ■ Relative defect □ Absolute defect

Visual field changes with ethambutol treatment (a paraxial optic neuropathy; b axial optic neuropathy)

B. Changes in Pupillary Function, Refraction, and Accommodation

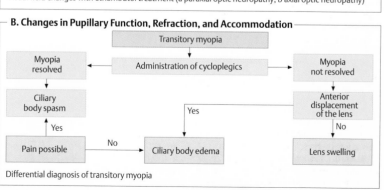

Transitory myopia

Myopia resolved ← Administration of cycloplegics → Myopia not resolved

Ciliary body spasm

Anterior displacement of the lens

Pain possible —Yes→

—No→ Ciliary body edema

—Yes (Anterior displacement of the lens)

—No→ Lens swelling

Differential diagnosis of transitory myopia

233

A. Epidemiology

The World Health Organization (WHO) in 1998 estimated the number of blind persons worldwide at 45 million and the number of persons requiring assistance because of impaired visual function at 150–180 million. Nine out of ten blind people live in developing countries; 60% of those affected are in Africa (south of the Sahara), China, and India. Eighty percent of cases of blindness are regarded by the WHO as avoidable. The most common cause of blindness is cataract, accounting for ca. 40–50%. Other diseases are trachoma, glaucoma, vitamin A deficiency, and onchocerciasis (**A**).

B. Cataract

The WHO estimates the number of persons blinded by cataract at 16 million. Age-dependent mature cataract (**B**) is the most common form of cataract. The fact that no surgical treatment is available to those affected or that the operation is not within their means is responsible for the large proportion of persons blind because of cataract in the developing countries. Various organizations have set themselves the goal of reducing the number of cases of blindness worldwide by half from 1999 to 2020 through the Vision 2020 project. This means primarily increasing the number of cataract operations in these countries.

C. Trachoma

Etiology/pathogenesis. Trachoma is an infection due to Chlamydia trachomatis.
Epidemiology. The pathogen is distributed worldwide and causes 15% of all cases of blindness. About 146 million persons require treatment. Trachoma occurs mainly in poor rural regions in Africa, where the pathogens are transmitted within families (finger-eye-finger).
Clinical features. Trachoma manifests itself primarily as keratoconjunctivitis with reddening of the conjunctiva, itching, and epiphora. The subsequent course of the disease is divided into five stages:

I   Follicular inflammation: there are at least five follicles on the upper tarsal conjunctiva with a diameter of at least 0.5 mm. Serous conjunctivitis.

II   Marked follicular inflammation: there are innumerable follicles on the upper tarsal conjunctiva. The conjunctiva is severely reddened, rough, and thickened.

III   Scarring after bursting of the follicles on the tarsal conjunctiva (**Ca**).

IV   Lid deformity because of the scarring. Trichiasis, with at least one lash rubbing on the eye.

V   Corneal opacities and reduction in vision (**Cb**). Severe scarring of the upper conjunctival fornix. Pannus formation.

Diagnosis. Clinical appearance. Histological evidence of the pathogen; culture or DNA evidence of the pathogen.
Treatment. Azithromycin.
Prognosis. The disease does not produce lasting immunity.

D. Glaucoma Diseases

Glaucoma comes third in the causes of blindness, after cataract and trachoma. Approximately 5.2 million persons worldwide are blind because of glaucoma, and glaucoma is suspected in about 105 million persons. Precise estimates are rendered difficult by the lack of a uniform definition of glaucoma and glaucoma diagnosis. Persons of African and Asian origin appear to develop open-angle glaucoma more often compared to caucasians. The disease is difficult to identify in the early stage because of the lack of symptoms. The treatment of open-angle glaucoma requires regular, often lifelong treatment with pressure-lowering eye drops. Alternatively there are various pressure-lowering operations (see Chapter 12). However, both conservative and surgical treatment are not accessible by or affordable for the majority of affected persons in developing countries.

A. Epidemiology

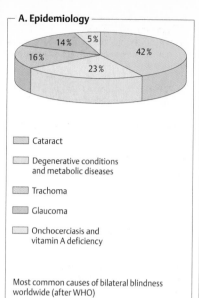

14 % 5 %
16 %
23 %
42 %

 Cataract

Degenerative conditions
and metabolic diseases

Trachoma

Glaucoma

Onchocerciasis and
vitamin A deficiency

Most common causes of bilateral blindness
worldwide (after WHO)

B. Cataract

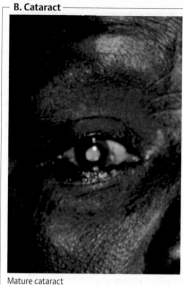

Mature cataract

C. Trachoma

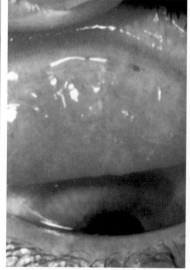

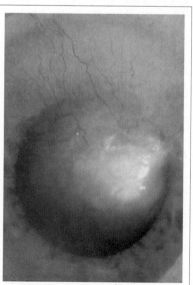

a Trachoma stage III

b Trachoma stage V

A. Onchocerciasis (River Blindness)

Etiology/pathogenesis. Worm infection due to Onchocerca volvulus. Female worms live parasitically for up to 14 years in connective-tissue nodules under the skin. They release microfilariae ca. 300 μm in size, which are taken up by the blood-sucking buffalo gnats and are transmitted to another human after formation of a larva.

Epidemiology. The pathogen is endemic in Africa and Latin America. It is estimated that ca. 18 million people are infected worldwide. Approximately 270 000 persons are blind from this cause, 99 % of them in Africa.

Clinical features. The microfilariae migrating through the body cause the clinical and especially dermatological symptoms. Adult worms lead to nodule formation. Blindness is the most severe consequence of the disease. If the microfilariae penetrate into the cornea or into the anterior segment of the eye, "snowflake" keratitis, iridocyclitis, neovascularization of the cornea, sclerosing keratitis with loss of vision, and blindness are seen.

Diagnosis. Clinical appearance. Microscopic detection in biopsies.

Treatment. Insecticides to control the buffalo gnat, which lays its eggs in rapidly flowing water. If the circulation of the disease is interrupted by 14 years, the reservoir of adult worms in the human population dies out during this period. Systemic treatment with ivermectin once a year.

Prognosis. Adult worms are not killed by ivermectin.

B. Loiasis/Loa loa

This is a form of filariasis caused by the nematode *Loa loa*. The disease is due to subcutaneous worms. The female subcutaneous worms are up to 7 cm long and the male worms up to 3 cm. The microfilariae released by the female worms are found in the peripheral blood and from there are transmitted to other persons by the sucking action of the horsefly *(Chrysops)*. The disease is endemic in the coastal countries of West Africa, especially in Nigeria and Cameroon. The principal manifestation is painful subcutaneous swellings on the distal limbs lasting 1–2 days (Calabar swellings) or involvement of periocular tissue. The symptoms are caused by the migrating worms. Subconjunctival motile worms can be seen under the slit lamp. The disease does not lead to blindness. Therapeutically the worm can be removed surgically. Diethylcarbamazine is available as a medication.

C. Leprosy

Leprosy is caused by *Mycobacterium leprae*. *M. leprae* is a very slowly replicating organism with a low risk of contagion. The disease occurs in tropical countries but is not linked to a warm climate. In 1996 the number of persons with leprosy was estimated by the WHO to be 1.3 million. The disease leads to blindness in ca. 50 000–100 000 persons. The clinical picture has two main forms, tuberculoid leprosy and lepromatous leprosy (transitional forms: borderline leprosy). In the tuberculoid form of leprosy, infection of peripheral nerves leads to the development of lagophthalmic keratitis with disorders of moistening and ulceration and thus to blindness. Keratitis and iridocyclitis are found in the lepromatous form. Systemic treatment is with dapsone.

D. Vitamin A Deficiency

Vitamin A deficiency leads to blindness in ca. 350 000 children annually. Vitamin A together with opsin produces the visual pigment rhodopsin and the cause of the disease is a dietary lack of the vitamin. Deficiency states lead to night blindness, dry conjunctivae (**xerophthalmia**), and the development of small gray-white plaques in the region of the palpebral fissure (Bitot's spots), keratomalacia, and ulceration. The deficiency can be eliminated by a high-vitamin diet or vitamin supplementation.

A. Onchocerciasis

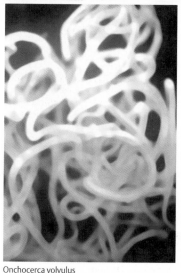

Onchocerca volvulus

B. Loiasis

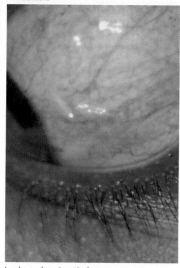

Loa loa, subconjunctival worm

C. Leprosy

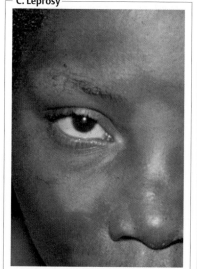

Lepromatous change in the face

D. Vitamin A Deficiency

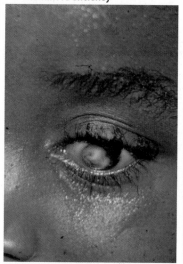

Corneal changes in vitamin A deficiency